Pit Banks to Red Benches

Pit Banks to Red Benches

From the Black Country to the Lords

By Jenny Tonge

Louisa Publishing

Copyright © Jenny Tonge 2021

All rights reserved. No part of this book may be reproduced in any manner whatsoever without written permission except in the case of brief quotations embodied in critical articles and reviews.

First printing 2021

ISBN 978-1-9196308-0-9

Louisa Publishing

This book is dedicated to my late husband, Dr Keith Angus Tonge, our children and grandchildren.

CONTENTS

Foreword
Prologue   African Mist   p1
Chapter 1   Childhood   p4
Chapter 2   Growing Up   p14
Chapter 3   Origins   p21
Chapter 4   Liberation   p26
Chapter 5   Following My Man   p33
Chapter 6   Into Politics   p43
Chapter 7   Honourable Member   p55
Chapter 8   International Development   p66
Chapter 9   Montserrat   p70
Chapter 10   Constituency Tales   p79
Chapter 11   Into Africa   p84
Chapter 12   Domes   p102
Chapter 13   The Poorest People on Earth   p109
Chapter 14   The Jewel in the Crown   p148
Chapter 15   Off the SCID   p154
Chapter 16   Big Smoke 9/11   p164
Chapter 17   Return to Africa   p169
Chapter 18   Drums of War   p175
Chapter 19   The Unholy Land   p181
Chapter 20   Darkness   p207
Chapter 21   Lords and Ladies   p214
Chapter 22   Coalition Blues   p219
Chapter 23   Chair of Pop and Sex   p223
Chapter 24   The Great Abortion Debate   p230
Chapter 25   FGM and Child Marriage   p236
Chapter 26   Better Off Dead   p241
Chapter 27   Epilogue   p245
Acknowledgements   p251

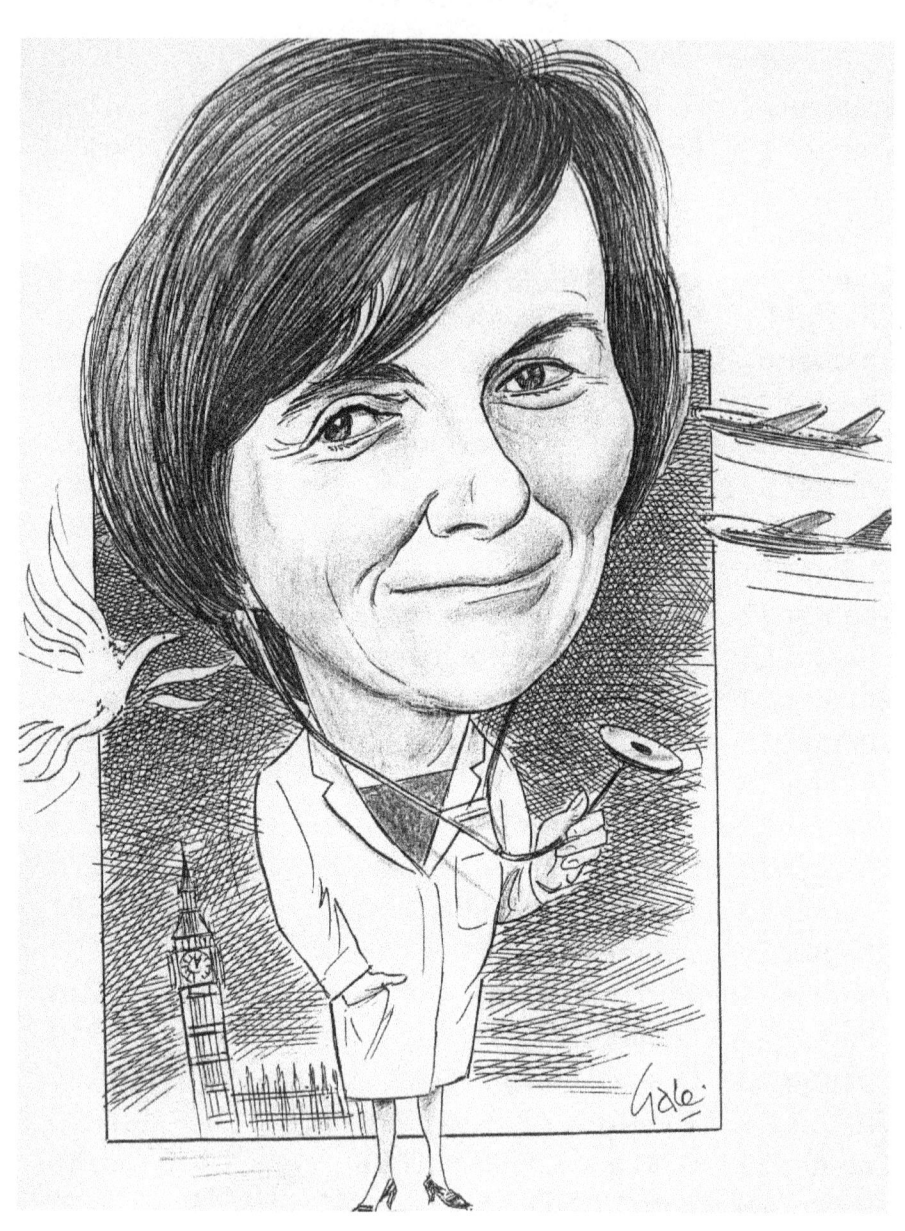

Jenny Tonge MP, by George Gale (1929-2003)

Foreword

I was never fortunate enough to serve in the Commons with Jenny Tonge – she arrived at the election where I left after 32 years, and I share her puzzlement that she was never given the Health spokesmanship for our party. But her position as our representative for International Development turned out to be a great blessing, well reflected in this volume of memoirs.

Her descriptions of her travels and encounters in so many poor parts of our world are laced with humanity and good humour, as is her obvious devotion to her Richmond constituency. That, combined with her life-long medical passion for family planning, is her lasting legacy, and I was fortunate enough to see her in action in the House of Lords and make one memorable visit with her to Sri Lanka.

As for her devotion to the Palestinian cause, she is absolutely right to remind us of the second part of the Balfour declaration, since largely ignored. I visited Gaza shortly after the "Cast lead" ghastly operation and share her revulsion and commitment to the downtrodden Palestinians. And if her language has not always been superbly diplomatic – so what; we have quite enough of that!

This volume will be of lasting interest, especially to her grandchildren, and it must be a real regret that Keith did not live to see it, nor continue to enjoy the little homestead by a river they had built together in the Languedoc, which Judy and I were lucky enough to visit.

David Steel, Baron Steel of Aikwood. KT, KBE, PC

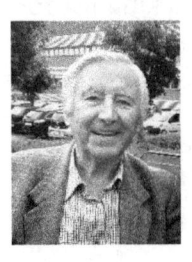

Liberal/Liberal Democrat MP for Roxburgh, Selkirk & Peebles 1965-83, Tweeddale, Ettrick & Lauderdale 1983-97
Liberal Democrat MSP for Lothians 1999-2003
Liberal Chief Whip 1970-76
Leader of the Liberal Party 1976-88
Presiding Officer of the Scottish Parliament 1999-2003

Prologue: African Mist

It was cold, with a thick mist swirling about, almost like a summer morning in Wales. We had been climbing gently up the mountain through dense vegetation to meet up with the guides for the morning. It wasn't Wales; it was Rwanda, near the Equator. We had come hoping to see the famous mountain gorillas, near the border with Congo – still a dangerous territory, with roaming militia groups from Hutu and Tutsi tribes always seeking one another out following the genocide years before in Rwanda. I was in there with a small party of MPs under the auspices of the Inter-Parliamentary Union.

Suddenly in the next clearing, there they were. It could so easily have been a human family resting after Sunday lunch. Father, the silverback, was sitting on a tree stump looking irritable, mother to his right with baby at the breast, a toddler playing at her feet and a 'teenage' gorilla larking about the group, clearly the source of father's irritation. Dad just wanted a bit of peace to contemplate the jungle. These were mountain gorillas, a protected species, hence the guides and wardens employed to protect them. Even so, poachers hunt and kill them, mainly for their meat.

They were enormous: broad, bulky animals with a strange, almost cross-eyed look; not benign, contemplating infinity like cats, but a strange, hostile, unreliable gaze, which said 'You are here at my pleasure, so beware'. We gazed – and I trembled a bit, I must say. We had been warned to stay quiet on meeting a gorilla and freeze if one charged us. We had been assured that they would not harm us. Easier said than done. I was glad that I had borrowed a jersey from one of the guides – jerseys hadn't been on my packing list for Rwanda. Anyway, I hoped the guide's smell would be less likely than my Madame Rochas to make Father Gorilla suspicious.

The teenage son was getting closer and closer to his father, flicking vegetation up at him and darting away. Father bared his teeth and issued a few warnings before becoming fed up with the teenager and charging at the group of us who were witnessing his humiliation. He stopped half way and stood glowering at everyone, human and gorilla.

There followed a curious dance between a Tory colleague and me, which would have been wonderful, slowed down, as an action replay. We knew we should freeze, but it was scary, and I slipped behind him for protection, and he immediately slipped behind me – a movement we executed a couple of times. Intrepid Oona King stood quite still with her camera and won all sorts of praise from the guides, whilst my other colleague and I found a tree big enough to shield us both. Just as suddenly, Father Gorilla changes his mind, gives us a disdainful glance, snarls at the teenager and returns to his tree stump. Mother looks up, sighs, and refrains from commenting on events. She shakes the baby round to her back and fends off the toddler, who by now was looking for protection in case Dad lost it. We stayed behind our tree for a few more minutes before Father decided the visitors, MPs or not, had been given enough chance to take photos. He strode off into the forest, followed by his obedient family, to try and find a better picnic spot away from the intruders.

The mist had now cleared, and sitting on the mountainside, watching the morning develop, I realised we were looking towards the Congo. I wondered how far it was to Lambaréné, in what was once French Equatorial Africa, where Dr Albert Schweitzer had set up his mission hospital in 1913. It always amuses me to think that it was a teenage crush on Schweitzer, which made me change O Level courses from Arts to Science to aim for medical school. I was a real geek at 14. Schweitzer was a Mother Teresa figure in the 1950s and had been a famous musician and theologian before giving up a stellar career to become a missionary. He had the same status as football heroes have with my grandsons now. He has been thoroughly debunked by commentators since, as paternalistic and a stubborn colonialist. Nevertheless, for me, he was a hero.

Reading his book now about his experiences in Lambaréné is a fascinating exercise. *On the Edge of the Primeval Forest* by Albert Schweitzer is a period piece written by a man who deplores the effect of colonisation on Africa and yet still has an incredibly superior attitude to the Africans. 'We all get exhausted,' he says, 'in the terrible contest between the European, who bears the responsibility and is always in a hurry, and the child of nature who does not know what responsibility is and is never in a hurry.' This last is an early reference to 'Africa Time', which we all recognise. My favourite comment from the great man is what he called his 'formula' – 'I am your brother it is true, but your elder brother.' He must have known what the Belgians had got up to in the Congo in the name of civilization and how they would lay down the administration which enabled the genocide in Rwanda to take place a century later. What problems he would have today! Were all we Europeans in a hurry when we colonised Africa?

Nevertheless, I decided I would do medicine because of Schweitzer, to my parents' delight, who were both school teachers and keen for my brothers and me to do academic things. A daughter as a doctor would be the heights in our little Black Country community in the fifties.

Chapter 1: Childhood

One of my fondest memories of my Black Country childhood was the railway cutting at the top of our road, which is an unlikely place to start a story. I often think of how we used to rush up the road, cross over the main road at the top and lean over the wall to see the train approaching. Noise, fire, steam, brimstone smells and lots of smoke in those days. Delicious. I can still smell the smell and sense the loss of street and buildings into the smoke for a while. I would cling onto that grey, flinty wall and dream of handsome princes and goblins or a glamorous grownup me doing exciting things. Maybe when the smoke cleared, it would be a changed world, to countryside or seaside, instead of the dark satanic mills in Tipton – my part of the Midlands. It was called the Black Country in those days and still is; black because of the heavy industry, mainly iron and steel foundries and the furnaces that put the 'great' into Great Britain in the nineteenth century. It is said that when the Royal Train carried Queen Victoria through the Black Country on her way to Balmoral, she insisted that the curtains of the train were drawn so that she did not have to look at the filth and squalor in which people lived. True or false? I don't know, but it was still an ugly area when I was a child.

I was a war baby, conceived in the Blitz and born as bombs rained down on the industrial Midlands early in 1941. My mother loved to tell me the story when I was in my teens and 'knew' about such things that whilst calling her two little boys in for tea one day, she suddenly realised that she had not had a period. Since when? When she realised it was far too long and must mean pregnancy, she worried that it would be a terrible thing to bring another baby into this world wracked by war, and England soon to be invaded by Adolf Hitler. Eldest sister Florence was consulted and said not to worry because a hot bath and as much gin as she could drink would 'start' her period. Gin was always known as 'Mothers' Ruin', of course. She would then say happily that not only did it not work, but she gave birth a few months later to a baby girl who grew up to have a lifelong love of gin. That was my beginnings.

There was a huge iron foundry about a mile from our little house, which opened its furnaces around my bedtime, or at least before I was asleep. I could see from my bed the red glow in the sky getting more and more intense and golden sparks like shooting stars lighting up my bedtime. It was almost worth going to bed for. In the days before health and safety regulations, we were taken as schoolchildren around another iron foundry to learn about industrial processes as part of the chemistry curriculum. I remember vividly being told to be careful while treading over one gulley full of cooling iron still at umpteen degrees Fahrenheit. No guards, no fences! The parents of most of my friends either worked in schools or in jobs connected to heavy industry or the car industry.

Manual workers still lived in tiny terraced houses. A row of houses near us that had escaped Hitler's bombs were called 'back to back'. Each house had one room downstairs and one upstairs, and the adjoining house behind was the same. Washing people and clothes was done communally 'out the back', where the lavatory was. Cooking and living went on in the downstairs room, and sleeping for the children was upstairs. Presumably, mums and dads liked a bit of privacy, especially when procreating. I often went into those places and wondered at the neatness and order that prevailed in most of them. My family house was a small three-bedroom semi, built on reclaimed pit land that my parents bought when they got married for a few hundred carefully saved pounds. Decades later, when my mother sold the house, the buyers' surveyor discovered an unfilled mineshaft just outside the living room window, where my father had put an Anderson shelter for us all during the war. We all gave thanks that no bombs ever came near enough to destroy the shelter and send us all down the mineshaft.

My parents were both schoolteachers and earned a bit more than the foundry workers whose children they taught. We had a long back garden full of trees and flowers, a different world from the front of the house. Lucky me – I used to lie under the small copper beech tree in that garden and look at the sky beyond, marvelling even then at the contrast between those shiny leaves and the translucent blue of the sky and wondering if any artist had ever managed to capture the contrast between them. The borders were filled with old-fashioned plants like pyrethrums and scabious and those big yellow daisies with black centres. The fences bore Paul's Scarlet and Emily Gray varieties of roses.

Further up the garden, there were rose bushes and tall delphiniums backed by the shrubbery beyond, where there was an apple tree and, from time to time, vegetables. My aunt's garden next door was much more practical. She liked to grow as much food as she could, and I used to help her pick blackcurrants with their musty, dusty smell. I loved doing that, much more than helping my husband on his allotment decades later – but then I had other duties too. I can remember every detail of that garden much more clearly than more recent things, which I know is an ominous sign as a doctor.

In those days, our bit of the Black Country was a real village called Ocker Hill, part of Tipton, named from the yellow ochre which used to be mined there long ago before the coal. The teachers and doctors, and in fact all professionals, lived in the area, unlike now with our ghettos for the middle classes. There were some between-the-wars council houses, which improved the living conditions for many people, but one area was notoriously called the 'Lost City'. People always referred to coming from 'up the Lost City'. It had no bus or rail connections and still hasn't as far as I am aware. I had two older brothers and several cousins who lived locally. Families still stayed close in those days. My father's sister and my favourite aunt, Aunt Ivy, lived next door, and I used to be allowed to sleep over at her house. I always had a candle night light beside my bed, resting in a saucer of water in case I knocked it over. Aunt Ivy was a tiny bird-like character with very twinkly eyes and a great love of children. She would tell me stories of my family and lots of nonsense too. She was wonderful and special, and I was born on her birthday.

Our social lives revolved around the church and the chapel, and never the twain would meet. We were 'church', and I did not have any friends from the 'chapel'. The two places of worship invited each other to services and festivals, of course, but we hardly ever went. The big thrill of the year was the Sunday School Festival. This was where rivalry really kicked in. We practised new hymns for the service to perform from the choir stalls on Festival Day. Such a thrill to be up in the chancel, which only my big brothers knew because they were in the choir.

We had new dresses for the festival, if we were lucky, made from hand-me-downs or cut down mums' things. My most memorable dress was the one my mother made from parachute silk. She and her sisters had clubbed together to buy a whole or half parachute from some postwar offer or other. The dress still had the parachute's seams running diagonally across the skirt, but my mother had smothered it in embroidered flowers. Oh, how I loved that dress. What skill my mother and most mothers had in those postwar years to create something out of nothing. The dress was worn proudly in the procession around the parish, which always took place on Sunday School Festival Day, preceded by the cross borne by church servers and choir and the Vicar in all his best robes. What a show! The Sunday school in their best frocks followed, and then the Scouts, the Cubs, the Guides and the Brownies, and finally the whole congregation, which was mainly men because the women stayed home to cook the Sunday lunch which even in those deprived days was still the main meal of the week.

On reflection, I think the primary purpose of all this pomp was to show the chapel people, who had a lesser procession the next week, that we were the top Christians. Chapel folk were often talked about in hushed tones. The nearest Catholic church was over a mile away and on another planet as far as we were concerned— such a narrow existence.

The main event of the year was the church nativity play, produced and directed by Vicar Bell's wife. I never got beyond being a baby angel, which may have suited me then, but it is not how I have turned out. I think my brothers were shepherds: one of them had a beautiful treble voice and always sang the choir's solos. And I seem to remember my mother being a shepherd too. Our Guide captain was the Virgin Mary. I used to speculate as to what the criteria were for being Mary, not having a clue about virginity at that age. My parents were in the dramatic society locally and did quite a bit of acting. Church activities coloured our lives, and I was glad I was 'church' and not 'chapel'. Now I am nothing really, thank goodness, but I still love the church liturgy and often go just to sit and meditate to the familiar words and music.

My friends and I all went to the local infants' school in Ocker Hill, where the milk was warmed in front of the classroom gas fire until playtime when we were forced to drink the disgusting stuff. I still have an aversion to anything milky and warm. That milk was in a small bottle and grew a thick skin during the morning, which broke the straw we were given. We were not allowed another and had to drink the foul stuff from the bottle.

One of our teachers had plaited hair wound into two buns, one on each ear. Her teeth were black, and she kept her handkerchief tucked into the elastic of her knickers. We all nudged and giggled when she went behind her tall desk to retrieve it. We learned by rote and us 'clever' ones, Brian Humphries, Betty Lyons, Ian Kennedy and me, sat in the front row and at reading time, we had to help the others. Ian Kennedy outshone our quartet in later years, being knighted after an illustrious legal career and a not very popular term sorting out MPs' expenses. I still see him from time to time, and we recall not just that classroom, but the nursery run by his mother that we attended in the war years, where we lay in little camp beds for our afternoon rest but spent most of the time whispering to each other. The discrimination between the clever kids and the not so clever kids was painful, but we somehow accepted it, I hope with good grace – probably not.

Those early post-war years were happy. The Attlee government made sure somehow that we had enough to eat – but not too much. Sweets were rationed, of course, and we raced to Mr Gittings' Sweet Shop on Fridays with our precious family coupons. We were allowed three 'quarters' of sweets for our family of five for a week—twelve ounces in all. We usually had mint imperials, a toffee thing and boiled sweets—something my children never had. We were spoilt. We brought our prize home and carefully shared each bag into three piles for my brothers and me. Any odd sweets were given to our parents. They had usually gone in a day, and the long wait started until next Friday, but that sensation of a hard toffee softening sweetly against my palate and slipping down my throat was bliss.

Fruit was plentiful in our family. My father knew someone out towards Evesham who allowed us to pick apples, and our garden had a Bramley apple tree. Did anyone else eat slices of Bramley apples which were accompanied by a minimal amount of sugar in a saucer to dip them in? As a grandmother, I have wickedly introduced my grandchildren to this delight when something sweet is called for.

My mother came in one day from the greengrocer and called us all in from the garden to show us this strange fruit we had only read about—the Banana. I later referred to it in a speech in the House of Commons on the banana trade as the 'original convenience food, hygienically packed and unwrapped easily to reveal a feast'. I could write an ode to my first banana.

Most tradesmen delivered in those days. The greengrocer, baker and butcher were the most frequent and welcome because their horses left valuable steaming manure on the road, which the men would rush out and collect for their gardens. Even more exciting was the coal man. He had a lorry and tipped the coal on to the pavement where we all muscled in to get it into our coal shed before it rained. Everyone helped and got filthy, which meant extra stoking of the fire for hot water to get us all clean before bedtime.

Saturday evenings were the highlight of the week because, if fine in the summer, we would go out to a country pub which allowed children in the garden to have 'pop' and crisps whilst our parents had a beer.

In winter, we would go to my father's youngest sister, who was married to Uncle Charlie, who had a newsagent's shop in Aston Lane, Birmingham. They were so kind to us. Uncle Charlie used to let me serve newspapers to his customers when I could just see above the counter, and by closing time, my fingers were black and shiny from the newsprint like his! That was a badge of honour. My brothers, meanwhile, if they were with us, went upstairs to gossip and play with our cousin.

Sometimes we all met my mother and aunt back there after we had been to watch 'The Baggies', West Bromwich Albion, play at the Hawthorns, also with Uncle Charlie. He always had a bottle of cold tea which we shared. Children sat cross-legged on the grass at the front – a far cry from football matches today. My favourite sporting memory came back to me last Christmas. I wake up very early since my husband died and immediately nearly fall out of bed as I reach across to turn on my radio and tune in to Radio 5 Live if a Test Match is on. Cricket from Australia sends me right back to childhood. (These early morning gymnastics have now been abolished by a Christmas present of a 'Google Home' which obeys commands).

As a small child, I used to patter into my brothers' room in the wee small hours, climb into bed with my eldest brother and snuggle down to listen to the cricket from Australia until stumps were drawn or it was time to get up. He had rigged up a loud speaker via curious cables up the stairs from the massive 'wireless' we had in the living room. I never knew why it was called 'a wireless' for that reason. The commentary waxed and waned and was always accompanied by the swishing sounds, which my brother reckoned were the waves in the sea on the way over to England. My other brother was a keen cyclist, and we used to pile into our little car to go to strategic points on his route to cheer him on, until one day, my father forgot to release the hand brake as we tracked him down a hill and the car ended up streaming smoke, and we had to wait for a tow home.

I played with my friends on bomb sites and abandoned pit banks. The bomb sites allowed the boys to throw stones at half-destroyed buildings and finish off Hitler's work. Nobody stopped us. It was a great release of energy, which children today simply lack. The pit banks behind our houses were grown over with patchy grass, and coltsfoots in spring used to provide bunches of flowers for the teacher that were put in fish paste jars.

The most significant event on those pit banks happened one day when I was out there with a younger cousin who lived near us – families stayed close in those days. A man approached and asked me to show him my knickers. I remember thinking he must be a bit odd and said I would do no such thing and sent my cousin off on his bike to fetch his mother, who lived very close. The man leapt on his bike and rode away. He had met his match. How did I instinctively do the right thing?

It did not put me off those pit banks. They were another world. When it rained, little rivers flowed down them, and we messed and marvelled for hours. The earth was grey, mixed with coal, and very bare. There was a disused canal too from the days when Tipton was a village and was described as 'The Venice of The Midlands' because we had more waterways than roads. The main remnant of those days was the big house where my friend Eileen Osborne lived with her father and mother. The house was attached to an office and staging post of the BCN, the British Canal Network, and he was the custodian of one of the Watt engines which used to pump water in and out of the canal system. It was housed in a unique building that was locked. Only special visitors were allowed into that hallowed space. Apart from the big main canals, there were lots of backwaters which, bar the odd dead dog or bedstead flung away, were a source of delight to us children. Tadpoles galore in the Spring brought home in jam jars carried with a string handle, sticklebacks and waterweed, and sometimes a bullrush or water iris. Treasures like that were fought over to take back to our mothers.

Our teacher parents always ensured we had a holiday every year. We had a Morris Eight car which took us everywhere. I sat on the back seat held between my big brother Michael's knees to stop me from lurching about. As we got older, the load became too much for our little car, especially on our frequent trips to North Wales, and when we got to a steep hill, everyone had to disembark. My father then drove up the hill while mother and children toiled up on foot to meet him. That was travel in the Forties! It took the whole day starting early to get from Tipton to Barmouth, less than 100 miles away.

At Easter, we went to wherever the National Union of Teachers held its conference, my father being a local official. It was usually at Scarborough, or those are the ones I remember because it always seemed to be cold, and we spent hours shut out of our boarding house during the day, not being able to afford hotels, and walking the freezing promenades and gardens of the place. I have never been back in adult life, so dire was my experience. Landladies really did not expect their guests to use the place except for breakfast and evening meal. Fondly remembered by my brothers and me too were the odd places that had pieces of newspaper strung together for toilet paper, which, as things gradually got better after the war, graduated to harsh scratchy stuff, one brand being called 'Bronco' I recall. It must have been difficult riding a horse after using that stuff every day!

Our summer holiday was usually chosen for the educational opportunities offered. My parents were teachers, after all, and liked to give us experiences. I consequently have visited and loved most of the cathedrals in England and keep vowing that one summer I will do nothing else but visit them all again.

My father always had a story to fix places in our mind. Did you know, for instance, that wicked King John is buried at Worcester Cathedral, and some hundred years ago they opened his coffin to confirm this? They were only able to catch a glimpse of the dead king because contact with the air made him turn into dust. It was a thrilling yarn for us children, whether it was true or not, and a fitting end for a king we regarded as bad, more because of Robin Hood stories than his mismanagement of the kingdom leading to the Magna Carta.

We were the fortunate ones. Many of our school friends had a trip to the local park to look forward to in the holidays, or two or three weeks 'hop picking' down in Kent, which was frowned upon by our parents and all our teachers because it continued into September and the children missed school. It sounded fun, though. They went in what were fondly known as 'Sharas', that is, charabancs, or coaches, to the southerner. It was like camping but with a bit of work thrown in and little supervision from parents because they were hard at it trying to earn money from the weight of hops they picked. Teachers were also very sniffy about it because the children came back 'lousy', meaning they had head lice which spread to everyone in the class. Regular visits by the 'Nit Nurse' took place to shame the children who had them. So silly and so good that this no longer goes on but is regarded as an inevitable minor curse of childhood.

Chapter 2: Growing Up

Childhood in the forties and fifties was deprived of the lavish presents and exotic foods that we could only read about, but it was happy, and the Labour government, conscious of the need to protect the next generation with its fledgeling NHS, ensured we all had our fair share of nutritious food and vitamins. Cod liver oil, Radio Malt and orange juice were available at the Welfare Clinic, and our mother dosed us with them all. Foul fishy cod liver oil first, then Radio Malt to take the taste away, and then diluted orange juice to finish. Welfare Clinics were where people took their babies for ritual weighing and 'advice'. They also vaccinated against polio when an epidemic struck. I remember us all queuing outside the clinic for that. Unheard of now except in developing countries and getting much rarer there too.

The greatest event in my childhood, however, was not a single event, but it certainly coloured the lives of my brothers and me and has made me reflect on the differences between health services then and now. As a small child, I was prone to ear infections, which led to much poking of my ear by the General Practitioner (GP) and my mother to 'clean' it. They probably introduced more bugs than they eliminated. I spent many winter weeks off sick, usually in my parents' bedroom, where burning coals from the living room downstairs would be brought up by my father and put in the fireplace to take the chill off the bedroom. No central heating meant only the living room was heated in the evenings by a coal fire, which heated the water for bedtime washing and early morning if it was rationed properly. Yes, and there *were* frost patterns on the inside of the bedrooms' windows in the mornings as my generation wax on about!

At around the age of six, I started having unexplained fainting and fits, and everyone got very concerned about me. The GP referred me to a neurologist attached to the University in Birmingham. Very eminent, he was called Professor Cloake. I must add that the waiting lists for anything in the newly created NHS were so long as to be legendary, and my grandmother's savings were offered to pay for the consultations. I remember those sessions vividly. The great professor decided to treat me with 'electrolysis' to stop the fits. I lay on his couch, and the trolley was wheeled in. An ice-cold, wet cuff was wrapped around my upper arm, which was stick thin – I was a very sickly child. An equally ice-cold, wet plug was inserted into my affected ear, and a switch was thrown. All I can remember was a sharp tingling all over, followed by the entire room rotating around me for what seemed like ages. I would then be sick, and after a little rest, I would go home on the long bus journey to wait for next week's torture session. Despite grilling specialists in the field as a doctor myself, I have never discovered anyone who recognised this 'treatment'.

After the course of electrolysis, the great professor wisely decided it was doing no good, and I needed an ear, nose and throat surgeon. An interesting postscript to the great Professor Cloake is that years later, when fighting general election campaigns in Richmond, his nephew, a retired diplomat and local historian, John Cloake and his American wife Molly, were great supporters of mine, and they allowed us to use their house on the terrace on Richmond Hill as a committee room. I often shared memories of his uncle with him when we had a quiet moment.

Professor Cloake's decision to refer me to the ear, nose and throat people was a wise one because, by that time, I was off school almost all the time and very poorly indeed. I had what is called a radical mastoidectomy, which meant that the inner ear mechanism was removed, and the abscess that was developing in the temporal lobe of my brain was drained and dealt with. Cure! What is especially interesting is that in those days, when a child was admitted to hospital, the parents were sent home, not to be seen for at least a week, the rationale being that visits from parents upset children and delayed their recovery. I was so unprepared that after being taken by a nurse that evening to have half of my head shaved prior to surgery the next day, I asked if that was it and could I go home now!

Anaesthetics were administered to everyone through a mask, and the patient was told to 'breathe the scent'. I felt I was being suffocated and fought back only to be held down firmly by one of the porters. It was terrifying. For those next few days, I had to have 'dressings' which involved ether being dropped onto a pad over my face to make me unconscious enough for the packing to be removed from inside my head and replaced. I pleaded with them that I would be good and bear the pain if only they would not suffocate me first! But it was to no avail. Every morning for a week, the trolley would clatter down the corridor and into the room I was in, and the process would be repeated. In all of this time, I was flat on my back with my head fixed, looking at a cracked white ceiling.

One day during that week, I opened my eyes and saw not the ceiling but the face of our local priest, Vicar Bell. We all loved him. He used to wear a huge cloak to walk down the road after church and we little ones used to hold on to his leather belt under that cloak and Vicar Bell would walk with three or four lots of small feet apparently propelling him like a robot, accompanied by shrieks and giggles from us. I suppose today it would be regarded as child abuse! Oh, how we loved that man. To see him there in that ghastly hospital proved to my childhood brain, or what was left of it, that God really did exist, and he loved me. I think I cried a little during that visit. Whatever I did, two days later, my parents also appeared, and recovery began. The tortures stopped, and by the time I was discharged from hospital six weeks later, I no longer cared about whether my family was visiting or not. I was allowed to 'help' the nurses push trolleys around wards and marvel at the sights I saw. I remember one man with a hole where his nose should have been and another person with what seemed to be half a face. It was fascinating to a small child, but that was not where my interest in medicine started. By the time I got home, I never wanted to see a hospital again. I did, though, for months afterwards, but at longer and longer intervals when my mother took me on the long bus journey, half my head padded and bandaged to see the great man who had been the torturer in chief. Months later, I was a bridesmaid at my favourite cousin's wedding with a specially created headband to contain the padding over my ear and disguise the lopsided hairstyle, which must have heralded the revival of the Mohican.

It meant I missed school for almost a year with only sporadic attendances, supervised by my father, who was head of my primary school. Life gradually returned to normal. I stopped having fits and faints. I put on weight and grew rosy. My auburn hair shone, and so did school. Apart from missing the learning of tables which annoyed my teachers, my education was unaffected by my illness. However, it left me deaf in one ear for all my life, which has enabled me to survive night flights into Heathrow and teenage parties upstairs, as well as providing an excuse that I did not hear when I do not want to do something. Bliss.

Those well-meaning but relatively ignorant doctors of the postwar years saved my life, and I constantly reflect on the amazing changes which have occurred in medical and nursing practices over my lifetime. It also reminds me of how fortunate I was to have such caring parents who somehow combined running their family with full-time careers in education. I must have made my two big brothers unhappy, though. Their sick sister constantly restricted their fun for a few years, but they were pretty good about it.

My 'big' brother Michael was my protector and could always cheer me up. He saw the funny side of most things and kept the whole family smiling. He revelled in the radio, as I do, and would sit chuckling at the Goon Show. My other brother had been the darling little one until that third child arrived and rather took his place, especially as she was a girl and always sickly and clever at school— poor boy. I was not so clever as my brothers, though. Once I got to grammar school, Michael helped me with Latin and History, and the younger brother got me through A-Level Physics by introducing me to calculus and quicker ways of doing things. He was aiming at engineering, although he went into business eventually. He was delighted, however, in later life when his daughter sailed into medical school and beyond!

As I grew older, life became even more serious: school meant working and talk about the Eleven Plus loomed. It did not concern me too much. Because of ill-health, I had gone to the junior school where my father was head and could look after me. Not to be recommended. My friends and I passed the Eleven Plus with flying colours and were praised and applauded by the poor lesser mortals who had to join in this adulation. They were banished to Secondary Modern schools, one of my favourite cousins amongst them. Luckily a music teacher there spotted his musical talent, and he became a fine trumpeter, but it divided us so much. Our extended family was never the same after the odious Eleven Plus. Education Ministers, please note. Children must not be condemned so easily when they do not have the right academic skill at the right time. Two of my friends and I went from Primary School to Dudley Girls' High School, where our mothers had been before us. It was quite old for a girls' school in the Black Country, having been founded in 1881, no doubt for the growing middle classes in Dudley who could afford it. I loved that school. It had some wonderful traditions all geared, looking back, to giving us girls the skills and confidence we needed to succeed in a man's world.

Something which would seem laughable now is that we had one lesson a week called elocution, where we were taught to speak without a Black Country accent. Laughable, yes, but only recently, thanks to some comedians and actors, Lenny Henry, in particular, has it become mildly acceptable. We have a Black Country poet now, Liz Berry, who is superb and makes it sing! Nevertheless, in the early fifties, when I was at secondary school, you were better without it, and once a week, we giggled our way through 'how now brown cow' and 'round the rugged rocks the ragged rascal ran'. It is a very miserable accent, and we did well to have it modified. We performed Gilbert and Sullivan operas too in collaboration with the Grammar school. I played the lead in Iolanthe and am still in touch with The Lord Chancellor, David Alexander.

The girls at Dudley Girls' High School ran their own affairs. Every form elected its Form President at the beginning of each academic year. Form Council was held every week at the end of Friday's lessons, and anyone who had a proposal about school rules or uniform and who had a seconder could have it discussed at Form Council. If it was approved, it was then the Form President's job to take the proposal to the School Council at the end of each month. School Council consisted of all the Form Presidents and their deputies plus the prefects (all elected) and two staff representatives. The elected Head Girl of the school presided, and minutes, agendas and constitutions were the responsibility of the elected School Council secretary, a post I held for two years. I would have preferred to be Head Girl because that was great and glorious, but I got beaten fairly in the elections and probably learned a lot more about how democracies are run as a consequence and how to show more humility in my dealings with other people.

This system had been running since the twenties when my mother was at the school and could change any school rule that we liked. The governors of the school had always insisted that the Head had a veto, but it had never been used and was not used when I was there. Women and girls, when they debate together calmly and sensibly, frequently come up with decent and workable solutions. How much better, I used to think; the world would be if it was run by women and not men.

The academic standard was good but not at the level of some schools nowadays, and the Head insisted on certain things. If we were to take a subject at A-Level, we did not take it at O-Level because that was regarded as a waste of time. Maths and English Language were always taken at O-Level, though. We did not get long strings of O-Levels, just the essentials for our future. I ended up with five O-Levels and six A Levels. Three girls in my year did A-Level physics and, because our school did not teach physics to A-Level, we had to go to the Boys' Grammar School twice a week to join their classes. No fun at all. The physics master was a monster who walked around the lab dictating notes which we had to take down and learn. The old adage of lecturing being the transfer of notes from the notebook of the lecturer to the notebook of the student without going through the brains of either was never more true. The most interesting part of his interminable drone was one particular gas tap on which he always caught his gown as he marched around us. Each time it tore a bit more, and I used to wonder when the gown would be torn off his back.

I had my little triumph with this man, though. Every week we had a test, and after a pretty awful mechanics week, the test was to derive the moment of inertia of a flywheel. Some readers may know what this is – I have never discovered it, but I do remember it took up two and a half pages of an A5 exercise book. We all groaned and did our best. The monster appeared, grinning in a sinister fashion, at the next lesson, and said that no one had had a clue and we must come back on Saturday morning for another test. We groaned and accepted our fate. I reckoned after some thought that he would probably just repeat the same question – just to trick us. So, I learned the dreaded derivation like a parrot and trotted it out when, just as I had thought, he repeated the same question on Saturday morning. The boys groaned, and I set to work before it disappeared out of my brain forever. Monday came, and he announced that everyone had failed the test yet again, except for Miss Smith, and her success was more due to her grasp of psychology than knowledge of mechanics. Triumph. He did respect us girls a bit more after that incident, though.

My beloved Dudley Girls' High School no longer exists, having been merged into the boys' grammar school (founded by Edward the Sixth) to form one big comprehensive, Dudley School. Long may it prosper. The two Dudley Grammar Schools had educated two generations of my family, and it was time to go.

Chapter 3: Origins

My mother, born Violet Louise Williams, came from very poor circumstances, from the striving working-class of Edwardian England. Her mother, Harriet, trained as a teacher and had fallen in love with and married George Williams, a foundry worker. He was what was described as a master moulder needed for the casting processes as molten iron came pouring out of the blast furnaces. Huge chains and anchors for ocean-going liners came from foundries like the one where George laboured. It was immortalised, I am glad to say, by the opening ceremony at the London Olympics in 2012.

Soon after the outbreak of the First World War, George had had a fiery argument with his employer and left to enlist in the army. Harriet, my grandmother, was left with five children and the proverbial shilling a day to support them. The stories from those times were legion. She had not worked as a teacher since her marriage, and she got by offering sewing services and sending one or other of the children to the pawnshop from time to time.

On one occasion, my mother had been told by the kindly pawnbroker that he could not bear to see my grandmother in such dire straits and that he would ensure that he and his wife would get enough sewing jobs for her and the girls to do to prevent other visits to pawn precious items. The Williams family kept a pig – many families did in those days – and the children of the family dreaded the day when 'Uncle Billy' came to slit its throat and butcher it into 'sides' to salt and hang over the winter. Chickens, too, supplemented the food supplies. My mother told me she had one with only one leg, which she pushed around on an old trolley pram that one of her brothers had made her. Somehow the family survived with occasional letters from their father, on one occasion apologising because the paper on which he wrote was badly torn due to a bullet having gone through his knapsack the day before. Reassuring stuff for the mother of five to endure back home. I still have those letters.

Miraculously George, my grandfather, survived the Battle of the Somme but was wheelchair-bound for the rest of his life. He could no longer work, but my enterprising grandmother managed to take on the franchise of the local public house and ran it superbly, cooking dinners for local workmen as well as ensuring the bars ran well. Grandfather and his wheelchair sat sternly in the bar and ensured respect and good order was maintained, or he would deal with it.

In later years, before my grandmother retired, as very tiny children, my cousin David and I used to creep into that same bar and sample the beer in the drip trays under the beer pulls until discovered by one of the aunts. Harriet and George managed to have one more child, Harry Aston Williams, who became a much-decorated bomber pilot in the Second World War. Being much younger than the rest of the family, he became like an elder brother to us, and when he came back after being a prisoner of war, he became part of our family. He and my mother won free scholarships to the grammar schools in Dudley, the one I attended years later. My mother said that when he was training in the RAF as a seventeen-year-old, he used to promise to fly over our back garden on sorties. Whether he ever did or whether we ever saw him, I do not know, but I do remember vividly as a child rushing into the garden every time we heard a plane, so novel were they in those days.

Violet Williams, my mother, fell in love with my father, Sidney Smith, who was also a teacher and son of the headmaster of the local school, where both families lived in Tipton. Sidney must have been quite a catch for Violet. His family were a 'cut above' hers, even if their origins were even more interesting. The story is that in the mid-nineteenth century, a traveller family passing through the Midlands called at a barrel maker's (cooper's) in Princes End, Tipton, to ask for whatever travellers of the day asked for. The barrel maker happened to remark on the fine family of boys and girls the traveller had, to which the reply came that there were far too many of them. Sadly, the barrel maker said how he longed for a boy to work for him, as he and his wife had no children. The traveller's father, it was alleged by Aunt Ivy, said he could have one of his fine sons. Whether money changed hands when the boy who was to become my great grandfather became the barrel maker's son is not recorded. Whether they were real travellers or not is a puzzle to this day. My aunt told wonderful stories, and I suspect the romantic Romanies of my dreams were actually just travelling tinkers.

You would expect that a tale of child slavery and deprivation would now follow, but the barrel maker and his wife were so delighted to have a child at last that the 'traveller' boy was treated as their beloved son and became Thomas Cooper-Smith. He was educated and taught the trade and grew up to inherit a very successful business. He became the Liberal leader of the local parish council and had several children, all of whom went on to higher education, this being quite an achievement at the end of the nineteenth century. One of those children was my grandfather, Thomas Smith. We all benefitted from the traveller and the barrel maker. The family have all tried to find out more about the travellers, but as we had inherited their family name of Smith, it became too difficult. Best just to dream of our origins and live with the genes we have.

My grandfather, Thomas Smith, was at University College London, my alma mater, for about a year but had to leave when his father died suddenly, and the remaining family needed him back home. He began to teach and became headmaster of the local Board School. His family of two boys and two girls were struck by tragedy when their mother, my grandmother, Agnes, died at barely forty and the eldest brother succumbed to meningitis a year later. Nevertheless, Aunt Ivy, my favourite aunt, took over the reins of the family and was adored by my father and his little sister. Intelligent, political, argumentative and kind, Ivy gave up education and personal gain for her family.

Sidney went to teacher training college because, yes, you have guessed it, his father died suddenly when Sidney was in his late teenage years, and he had to get his training finished quickly and start supporting what remained of his family. He taught in the local school where his father had been headmaster. Around this time, my mother had failed the French exam in her matriculation exams, and her ever-ambitious and resourceful mother had looked for a tutor to help her pass the second time, which she did. The tutor she employed was the son of the late local headmaster! My father fell in love and, despite a six-year age difference and allegedly being 'spoken for' by someone else, persuaded my mother to marry him.

Theirs was such a love story deserving of a separate book. In old age, my mother showed me a bundle of his letters and poems written to her, which she had kept with the message inscribed on the outside of the packet, 'Jen, read these when I am gone, and you will understand why there was never anyone else for me.' They were letters from my father over about two years trying to persuade my mother that there was no one else he loved and that she was not stealing him away from anyone else. She clearly needed a lot of persuading because the correspondence went on and on interspersed with poems he had written for her.

After my father died, my mother never really recovered her spirits. Strangely, we never found any of her letters to him, even when I was delegated to clear the desk in the headteacher's office he had occupied. Do men not keep letters? I guess they don't. It is just we women who treasure memories of loved ones in written form. At least, it seems to apply to my family. Anyway, their marriage had to wait. My mother was terrified to be seen as a hussy who had snatched him away from someone else – and she from the local pub too!

They were absolutely devoted to each other and to us, and our childhood was wonderful as a result, even if not especially well-off. Sadly, because he had died, in the time-honoured tradition of our family, he never knew I had gone to university, which he so wanted for me. Perhaps because of his mother's early death and the responsibility placed on his elder sister to look after the family, my father was fiercely protective of women's rights and always insisted that family chores were shared. He famously got us all up and dressed every morning and school books sorted whilst my mother cooked breakfast. He constantly impressed on me that I should take every opportunity early on to get qualifications because if I married and had children, I would have to lose time out of whatever career I was in to raise a family. Not many fathers had that attitude towards their daughters, although times were gradually changing as the war had once again made it almost essential for women to work outside the home in the absence of the men.

It is difficult to forget that summer day towards the end of the long holiday. I was sitting in the garden, chatting with my mother and my friend Eileen Osborne, when we heard a cry from the garage at the end of the garden where my father was sawing some rotten wood out of a support. We ran to the garage finding him confused and struggling to his feet. We somehow got him, half-walking, half-dragging, onto the lawn where he lay, protesting that he was fine but cradled in my mother's lap. I could not believe that my adored father was really ill.

I was sent to summon a doctor, and the long wait began. The doctor eventually arrived and decided that he should go to the hospital by ambulance, but as we progressed over the bumpy Black Country roads, he lapsed into unconsciousness, clutching my mother's wedding ring. This was something she never forgot, that even though unconscious and dying from a massive stroke, he was still holding her ring on her ring finger at the end. This became symbolic for her of their undying attachment, and of course, even though she was only 48 years old, she never remarried. I wondered too if I would ever marry. Surely it was now my duty to focus on a career to make my father's ambitions come true.

Chapter 4: Liberation

I went up to University College London (UCL) in October 1959, just a year after my father's sudden death. I was excited and apprehensive about going to university in London. My brother had borrowed his friend's beautiful old Riley car – with running boards! I sat in the back with the box containing the half-skeleton, which was on the list of needs for medical students in those days. Our local GP, who had cared for me throughout my childhood, had lent me his skeleton from his student days, so it was doubly precious. I had only visited London twice during my childhood, with the teacher parents always ensuring that every treat was fun but educational at the same time. That was a golden age for students. I did not have to give up or shorten my higher education for family reasons. The state not only paid my fees but as a fatherless student, I was awarded a generous maintenance grant for my entire five years of medical training. Thank you, UK taxpayers and a good government.

UCL was liberation. I was desperately homesick at first but soon began to enjoy the freedom of having no one to watch and advise and criticise. However, as my father had died so recently, I felt his presence often, and I think it kept me sensible. Medical student life in those days was hard academically but such fun.

I was a rugby club follower because most of my friends played the game. Wednesday and Saturday afternoons were devoted to the game and the consumption of beer afterwards. We girls went along if we were free. At one stage, I was honoured to be the kit mistress: I had a sewing machine, and so I was delegated to stitch numbers onto shirts. My duties extended to helping wash the same shirts in the student hostel basement after matches. I thought it was fun and was called 'one of the boys' as a consequence. Their other name for me, as a consequence of hauling kit about (helped by other girlfriends of the team), was 'the old bag'. You could not get higher accolades than that in the early sixties when our male-dominated society was just beginning to be questioned. University

College Hospital (UCH) was not a great rugby team because the UCL intake did not come in on rugby scholarships which was how, it was alleged, medical schools such as St Mary's Hospital and Guy's came to dominate the student rugby scene. Whether true or not, they produced good doctors! Maybe good doctors need more than brains?

UCL was founded in 1826, inspired by the ideas and philosophies of Jeremy Bentham, John Stuart Mill and others, to provide a university for people who did not belong to the Church of England, which was the prerequisite for Oxbridge. UCL was very special: it was known as the 'Godless Institution in Gower Street'. Soon afterwards, King's College was founded by the Anglican Church to provide a holier education for Anglican students in London. This formed the basis of the running but good-natured feud, which had persisted to this day as students. We derided King's as they derided us. Some students from King's College really did kidnap Charlie the stuffed ape, the mascot of our Common Room, and some of our students had to go and rescue him. It happened and was not just an invented scene in the film *Doctor in the House*.

There were 120 students in our year, only ten of whom were women, so we had quite a time of it. The student nurses in our year were also around socially, and we all trained and grew up together. We rubbed shoulders with students of all the other faculties, and we were not confined to medics, as were the students of the other medical schools in London. My dearest and closest friend is a historian who I met at UCL. I shared flats and digs and motherhood and retirement with Margaret (Maggie) McDougall. She is the nearest thing I got to have a sister, but with the added advantage of being wise counsel on many issues, especially putting modern politics into a historical context. She and her husband Robert Hurst went to live in France and reared their family there, which is why we eventually had a tiny house near a river in the Languedoc near them, now sold to a lovely young French couple. It had a meadow going down to a stony river, fierce in winter. A little wood grew up on half the land which my grandchildren called 'The Enchanted

Forest'. No princes there, though. It was my husband's dream to return to his farming roots in his retirement and be self-sufficient there. Sadly, he never made it.

I found the work of those pre-clinical years so difficult. Science A Levels had been bad enough for a girl whose favourite subjects had to be abandoned to do sciences for medical school entry. I remember going to the first biochemistry lecture at UCL given by Dr Prakash Datta, later to become Professor of Medical Biochemistry at UCL. I did not have any idea what he was talking about – a feeling shared, I am glad to say, by a number of our year. We decided he had done it to impress us and retired to our watering hole, The Lord Wellington, the students' local pub across the road, now named The Jeremy Bentham. We gradually warmed to biochemistry and at least saw its usefulness. We warmed to Dr Datta, who had never really stopped being a student and would arrive at medics' parties with something called 'Datta's Punch', which had some of our number legless by the end of the party.

The other, never to be forgotten experience, was our first day in the dissection room. Groups of six students were allocated to a dead body which we would then dissect for the next eighteen months for two sessions a week. With eyes often streaming from the formalin, the bodies were kept in between the ordeals in the dissection room. On our first day, six of us stood gazing at this dead man, who we called 'Albert', wondering if anyone would faint. We were, after all, fresh from school, no gap year and absolutely no talk to prepare us. Strangely, I do not remember thinking about my father, who had died only a year before, because what lay before us no more resembled a human being than a pickled onion resembles an onion plant! Nevertheless, it was by dissecting this man that we found out how the human body is constructed. There were no 3D computer images in those days.

After what seemed like an age of shuffling from one foot to the other and trying not to look too intently at Albert, a firm voice said, 'Shall we introduce ourselves? I am Keith Tonge.' This was my first encounter with the man with whom I would spend most of the rest of my life. No thoughts of romance then, though. We got down to the business of opening up the abdomen, guided by our dissection manuals, to see what was there.

Physiology, pathology, anatomy all followed in a mass of information we were supposed to absorb in less than two years before moving on to the wards to see patients and learn about illness. Somehow most of us passed the notorious 'Second MB'. Keith Tonge did so well that he was offered an extra grant to do a degree in biochemistry before embarking on clinical work. I managed to pass despite crashing part of my pathology viva, which stuck in my mind as an early example of discrimination. The outside examiner asked me all about food preservation, of which I knew little despite my mother bottling fruit when I was a child. I certainly had not expected to have questions on it. It was not, as far as I can recall, in our textbooks! The examiner remarked that I should know about these things because I was a woman. Red-faced and furious, I somehow found the right door and got out, sure that I had failed. Fortunately, I did not, and the home examiner assured me that not to worry; his colleague was always like that with the girls.

Keith Tonge made his mark early on when we were directed to attend our first post-mortem examination. The old post-mortem room was at the back of the hospital, and to get to it, we had to clamber up a flight of iron fire-escape stairs. The corpse arrived by another route, I hope with a little more dignity. I suppose we thought there would be another pickled Albert lying there, but there was not. What looked like a just-dead person was something quite different and very lifelike, if you can say that about a corpse. It was white and floppy with a sickly smell that reminded me of rotting lilies. It oozed as the pathologist made an incision into the abdomen, at which point we heard a crash and saw our colleague Keith flat on his back and unconscious. He later said it was the smell when he was endlessly teased about us having to drag him head first, down the iron stairs and into the fresh air. Luckily it was just a stone's throw from The Lord Wellington, where he quickly revived.

Sadly, I am left with a dislike of lilies which always remind me of the poor corpse and that day.

When we entered the portals of the great University College Hospital, we were allocated to medical 'firms', headed by a consultant of course; two or three junior doctors were the staff sergeants. We would line up each morning before ward rounds to be inspected for tidiness before the great man (there was only one woman consultant in those days) arrived, usually in a very smart car, at the doors of the hospital, to be greeted first by Matron and then on to his 'firm', all standing to attention.

Consultants usually reserved a pithy remark for the woman student on the 'firm'. We were tolerated as part of the march of modernity but not welcome. It really was like that. Nevertheless, I loved the clinical work. This is what I wanted to do, and being a woman, I could have so much more empathy with the women patients who were often not understood by the male medics. How can men understand what it is to be a wife and mother and also, in many lives, the provider too? It is called multitasking nowadays.

The years passed so quickly, and Keith and I became an 'item' in our year, together with other couples who had found their mates the same way. We smoked and drank merrily, that is until the Royal College of Physicians produced their report on smoking and lung cancer. We stopped smoking and stuck to beer. Until then, a night on call, when there was no point in going to bed, was spent in Night Sister's office smoking and drinking black coffee to keep us awake for the next emergency. Hours were spent under the hot lights of operating theatres, hauling on retractors to keep cavities open whilst the surgeon delved, trying all the time to keep our leg muscles moving so that we did not faint!

All medical students had to do two weeks acting as novice nurses on the wards, and here discrimination kicked in. I remember the boys being given medical type tasks to do, whereas we few girls made beds and emptied bedpans in the sluice like junior nurses did in those days.

Obstetrics should have been more fun, but I was sent to Nottingham to do my obligatory fifty deliveries. Here there were no friends, and it was a very dreary hospital and city in those days. The superintendent midwife was a dragon, a devout Christian, who I suspect would never have been recognised as such by Jesus of Nazareth. She refused to allow any painkillers for the young unmarried mums in labour because they must suffer for their sins. The consultants just shrugged it off as her eccentricity, but I hated that cruel woman and used to wish she could have a little experience of what she imposed on others. We also agonised over the disdain for women who had had illegal abortions and complications had set in. Some died, but there never seemed to be much sympathy for them. Much better was going out on a bicycle with the midwife on call to do home deliveries and sometimes having to call the 'flying squad' ambulance to take a mother into hospital with a frail baby or a post-partum haemorrhage. Those were the days.

Memories of the student days are beginning to fade except for three events that occurred when we were all together. One morning we woke up to the news that large white footprints had appeared all the way up the wall of the nurses' home, which backed onto the medical students' hostel. Matron was seriously affronted because, only a few weeks before, the nurses had woken up to find the entrance to the nurses' home had been bricked up by students during the night. Criminal proceedings had not followed, but the appearance of the feet must have been the last straw for her, and we imagined her stamping into the Dean's office to demand action. Certain members of the medical school were summoned to the Dean to own up or explain, with Matron present. They were given a severe dressing-down, and Matron was appeased. Once she had left, however, the Dean wanted to know how they had done it and who was the brave abseiler. He was one of our group but should remain anonymous. As far as I know, traces of those feet are still there.

Much more serious was the Cuban Missile Crisis, when we sat in the refectory most of the day waiting for World War Three to break out before the Russians turned tail. It seemed that day that nuclear war was imminent, and all would be lost. It seems crazy now, but it was very real then.

In our final year, my crowd were in my room having coffee – we took it in turns to do after-dinner coffee and chat before starting the big swot for finals. Howard Thomas, a Welshman and rugby captain at the time, came rushing in to tell us the news that President John F. Kennedy had been assassinated. We were all devastated. He was every student's hero in those days, despite his many faults. No work that night as we sat and talked about our future. That same student, Howard Thomas, has kept our year together well into retirement with annual reunions and messages. He now regularly spreads the news that yet another one of our year has died, whilst he tends his wife, who is severely paralysed after a massive stroke. He is a real hero. We all went our separate ways after finals. I loved phoning my mother after my finals and hearing the operator ask her if she would pay for a reversed-charges call from Dr Jenny Smith. She burst into tears! All her hard work and care, especially after my father died, had been rewarded.

I did not get a first house job at UCH. I was very disappointed and was told by my consultant boss, when I returned to UCH as a casualty officer a year later, that I had been instantly excluded because when I was asked what I was going to do in the few weeks before the jobs started, I had said quite truthfully that I was going to get married. How could a married woman take a house job seriously, let alone a whole career in medicine? I was instantly removed from the shortlist.

Chapter 5: Following My Man

It will seem very strange to young people now, and so it should, that having sex before marriage was a fairly risky thing to do with only condoms for protection – if that – and abortion was illegal. Consequently, I was pretty resistant to all temptation because I wanted to pass my finals and not let my mother down by getting pregnant. We consequently decided to get married and have a big party for all of our year group after finals. Interesting to note that on visiting a Marie Stopes clinic a couple of weeks before our wedding for contraception, with an engagement ring sparkling on my finger, I was told they could not help but to come back when I was married. How our society loved to control women.

I love the Marie Stopes organisation, and since that first visit, I have worked for them and seen their wonderful work all over the world. I did not realise that then. Our wedding, laid on by my proud mother, was attended by most of our medical school year who hired a coach to come to the Midlands to see us wed. We had great fun for a few years attending each other's weddings, which were still the only way most young couples managed to live together in those days.

We never lost touch with our 'year', so close a band we were. The most recent reunion, sadly, was the 60th year after qualifying. I am afraid I no longer go to them, having been 'denounced' as antisemitic in a letter to every member of the group by an Israel supporting colleague – with a deafening silence from the others. It was only refuted by one person who had worked in the West Bank and Gaza for several years. No one wished to offend, of course, but I felt I had to leave this charade and show them that I was not going to smile and carry on when such injustice and horror was being perpetrated in the Occupied Territories of Palestine, and they would not recognise it, for fear of offending members of our year and colleagues in the medical profession.

Evil triumphs, they say, when good men do nothing. I would add that friendship also survives anything if strong enough. It did.

After qualifying and marrying, we all went our separate ways, including Keith and me. I got a junior hospital job in the Midlands with a UCH trained cardiologist, and Keith went back to UCL to complete his clinical training after his BSc. We started our married life together a hundred miles apart except for the odd weekend when he would come and join me, and we squeezed into a sagging single bed in my doctor's residence room. Great fun. On hot nights, which were frequent, owing to the gurgling central heating pipes that ran up the wall by the bed, one of us slept on the floor. Such was the life of a junior doctor in those days.

The food, though, was amazing. The doctor's residence in the hospitals I worked in would cook proper fresh meals and a roast on Sundays. The cooks would bleep absent doctors and tell them they must come to be fed, and if impossible, it would have to be left covered up in the warm oven. We ate many a desiccated, once delicious, home-cooked meal in those days, but I still reckon it was better than the rubbish that is served up today.

My surgical job was at the West Middlesex Hospital in Isleworth, where on odd weekends off, I fell in love with the London Borough of Richmond upon Thames. For a Black Countrywoman, reared amongst the foundries and canals, Richmond seemed like an earthly paradise. I returned to UCH as a Casualty Officer, which was tremendous fun. There was never a dull moment in Casualty in those days. As students, we had done a month or so there. It was in the days of the Victoria Line construction, and we used to get totally exhausted, mainly Irish, men in Casualty with minor injuries, but also suffering from exhaustion. The conditions down in that tunnel were atrocious, but they worked with great good humour, and I think loved coming into Casualty for a bit of tender loving care. I was ordered to wash the feet of one guy whilst he was waiting to see the doctor. The formidable Sister Kirk, full-bosomed against all comers, if not the wind, liked us to be useful. As I peeled the boots and socks off his very cheesy feet and started to bathe them, he touched my hair and said, 'Doctor, you are just like Maureen O'Hara.' She was an Irish film star, popular at the time. I felt so privileged in a funny way to tend that man.

I also remember a young woman with vague abdominal pains and a missed period, who I left for a few minutes to get the registrar for advice. When I came back to her, she was losing consciousness rapidly, and her blood pressure was in her boots. It was an ectopic pregnancy, of course, and she was saved in the nick of time as we poured blood and plasma into her on the way to the theatre.

My greatest triumph in Casualty was to diagnose two dissecting aortic aneurysms over a two-week period. Aortic aneurism, as every watcher of TV medical soaps knows, is a very dangerous condition, and if it bursts, you die. It is as simple as that. My two patients were diagnosed by me, taking a good history and performing a proper medical examination, which never seems to happen nowadays. Patients now are sent off for tests and scans before being examined – or so it seems. The patients were rushed to the theatre and survived.

You can imagine my self-doubt and hesitancy when the following week, *another* man presented with abdominal pain. There were not many clues as to what was causing it, however, except rather a strong 'pulse' when I pressed on his very obese abdomen. Could it possibly be another? I decided to tolerate the mockery and over-cautiousness if I was wrong and once again called the registrar. This patient was observed for 24 hours and then was rushed to the theatre to have his aorta repaired. The Professor of Surgery had the good grace to come down to Casualty and thank me for my good work but remarked that it was probably due to female intuition more than anything else. I refrained from kicking him in a painful place. We women were used to being patronised. Grrrrr. How many times during my training did I wish I was male, not female, just to get treated with some sort of respect.

Quiet times in Casualty, usually during the night, were spent smoking and drinking in the kitchen and nodding off. Sometimes the local bobby on the Gower Street beat would join us. Gower Street was a sex workers' walk in those days, and they used to congregate at a sandwich and coffee van near the main road. I always felt so sorry for these girls and women who could find no other way of feeding their families but to sell themselves so dangerously. Many of them were my patients when I did home visits in Battersea years later.

After my time as a Casualty Officer, I became a Registrar in the Pathology Department, learning a little more about biochemistry and haematology with old friends like Mike Emmerson, our best man, who became an eminent bacteriologist, and Dan Thompson from our dissection table, who did equally great things in haematology. We were joined by the brilliant Peter Garcia Webb from Guy's. Most of the medical staff below consultant level were UCH trained, so it was brave of Peter to join us and eclipse the likes of me! He eventually became a consultant medical biochemist and emigrated to Australia, but such was the bond between us all from those hellish (for me) days in the lab that none of us lost touch with each other. It was a great crowd, but I hated being up in the lab and away from patients.

Doctors on the wards would order great batteries of tests out of hours and expect fast results. *We* never saw the patient except on one wonderful occasion when down a microscope, I had spotted meningococcus in cerebral spinal fluid from a sick child. He was the patient of the Sub Dean of the Medical School, one of the most human consultants around. Dr Bernard Harries came up to the lab in the middle of that night to seek me out and say, 'well done'. He took me down to the ward to show me the child I had 'saved'. Meningitis is deadly unless diagnosed and treated very quickly. That incident made pathology worthwhile, but not for long! Mostly it was slave labour on auto-analysers hissing away and running out of reagents at crucial moments. Ghastly work. No computers then, although the auto-analyser, I am told, heralded the computer age in pathology.

During this time, we had been living first in a flat in Golders Green, in north London, and then a flat in Islington purchased through a first buyer scheme from the Greater London Council on a 100 per cent mortgage. A brilliant scheme because it also prevented us from making a huge profit by selling on, because our reselling price was set by them. We decided after a year or so that we must try to buy a terrace house in Islington as my canny husband reckoned it would be a good investment. This led to another little brush with discrimination against women because we needed to borrow £5000. We trailed around banks and building societies to no avail because, even though we were both qualified doctors, Keith's salary was still low, and my salary could not be taken into account because I was a woman and would have babies.

We eventually found a kind manager at the local Westminster Bank, who agreed with us about a house in Islington being a good buy and agreed to lend us the money we needed. What a star! In grateful thanks, we both changed our accounts to the Westminster Bank, now NatWest, and despite their tribulations, have stayed with them as they stayed with us. It was the best decision we made in the early years of our marriage and meant eventually, as we moved around, that our children and we would always have roofs over our heads.

Our little house was in an early Victorian terrace, with no bathroom and an outside toilet. We worked hard all day, and when we were not on night duty, we tore paper off the walls, borrowed more money to build a bathroom at the back and generally make it habitable. We loved that house, even if everything fused when it rained heavily, and Keith had to go under the pavement to the 'cellar' in industrial gloves to reset the main switch. Once the house was ready, I became fed up with no patient contact in the Pathology Department, became pregnant with our first baby, David, and started doing GP surgeries for two sessions during the day and two evenings. We were desperately poor in those days. I linked up with another mum I had met in Islington, and we each worked two mornings a week whilst the one at home looked after the babies. Jane was the wife of an Oxbridge medic in our year who had seen the same potential in Islington and sunk their all into buying a house. There was no option – we women had to work to help the finances. I did evening surgeries too, and later on could be seen with baby ready for bed, waiting for husband to come home on his nights off to babysit whilst I worked. We had no holidays either for a few years, as Keith did GP locums in his holiday time. They were not very happy years. I found life very boring compared to hospital doctoring and missed our friends at UCH.

I founded a 'Pram Club' at the local church for similar lonely mums in the area, and that provided some fun, although they quickly latched on to me being a doctor and wanted advice about all sorts of problems. It also gave me great insight into the lives of poorer mums trying against the odds to feed and clothe their families in poor housing conditions. It filled the long hours between work and Keith coming home, which was not very often. He had chosen radiology as his speciality and was still in the teaching hospital environment having a ball. It was this slight boredom that led to the birth of our daughter Mary. It seemed to me that I might as well be bored and worn out by chores and surgeries with two babies, as with one. I was fortunate in having such lovely kids, though: they were not that much of a burden and, as they got older, became my pride and joy together with their little brother, who came much later.

After a few years, Keith got a very good senior registrar training post at the Queen Elizabeth Hospital in Birmingham. He was delighted, and so was I. It meant I could be within half an hour's drive of my mother and various members of my family. It did not escape my calculating mind that my mother was aching to have charge of her grandchildren for a few hours a week and that if I could find some medical work in the area, I could still get more experience in general practice and contribute to the finances. They were such happy years. We lived in rented hospital accommodation for a few months, watching our house in Edgbaston being built!

The Islington investment had paid off, and we moved into a so-called 'Gentleman's Residence' in a spaciously laid out cul de sac of new four-bed houses with two bathrooms and electricity which did not fail us in the rain – although it did fail us during the Ted Heath strike period when we had to cook by Calor gas camping stove. David and Mary had safe open spaces and trees and friends. They loved that place, although looking back, it was a bit posh for our Islington mindset, used to the terraces and early Victorian ethos in architecture and home decor. Keith called Edgbaston 'Gin and Jaguar Belt', although I suspect it was because we could still only afford a Morris 1000 Traveller, followed by a second-hand VW Combi to transport our brood. Our near neighbours thought we were rather strange for doctors! I don't know what they expected. A bigger car, perhaps? One of them became a close friend, though, and her two children became best friends with our two. I used to love to take the four of them out and have people think they were all mine.

It was here, with my mother's help, that I was able to train with the Family Planning Association (FPA), who were then the main providers of contraception. Men could always go into the local pharmacy and get 'something for the weekend', that is condoms, but women either had to talk to a GP, who might or might not prescribe 'the pill' which had been introduced in the 1960s or go for more expert advice at a family planning clinic, where they faced close questioning about their personal situation and a full medical examination before being prescribed the pill. I became incensed then, and still am, that the NHS, at that time, mostly male doctors, had control over the fertility of us women. Contraceptive methods were available, and in time most of them became far less dangerous than aspirin which we could buy anywhere. Nevertheless, the NHS doctors had to be seen before we could access contraception. Luckily for me in Birmingham, at that time, I was able to do the very thorough theoretical and practical training offered by the FPA - I even did their course in public speaking and how to give talks! I did not really need the latter because, thanks to my father, I had never been shy of speaking in public. In fact, I loved it. As a teenager, I had wanted to be an actress for a while and went from time to time on a train ride to Stratford on Avon to queue for the 'standing' tickets at the Memorial Theatre, which only cost ten shillings. I was besotted by the theatre but was dissuaded by my school from such notions because to do so would be 'wasting my God-given talents', by which they meant passing exams and going to university for the glory of my school. I contented myself with the school choir and annual Gilbert and Sullivan operas.

In my clinics in Birmingham, I learned the real difficulties faced by women, especially amongst the ethnic minority communities. The men came into the UK having been 'supplied' with a wife through the community network. The women, often only young girls, would come over to be married and not speaking a word of English had to rely, in the early stages, on their husbands accompanying them to see the doctor. Later on, they brought their children, who were rapidly learning English at school. It did not always help very much. One lady came back pregnant after being put on the contraceptive pill by a colleague. Her husband said he simply could not understand it because he had taken the pill regularly every evening! He came to no harm. Another patient, who had been given the cap to use by her GP, was having great difficulty because she lived with her extended family, with a shared sink on a landing and the only lavatory in the house being outside at the back. Those early years in family planning and sexual and reproductive health were invaluable for my future interests.

After four years, we were on the move again with Keith's career. He had taken up a job at the Royal Marsden Hospital to research breast cancer imaging, and after months of living apart once again, we managed to sell our lovely house in Birmingham and move back to that other 'smoke', London. At that time, Maggie McDougall was living in Kew with her family and suggested we might move there. I was very enthusiastic because of my six months in the area doing a house job at the West Middlesex Hospital. It was not easy, however. House prices in London had risen way above what we were used to in Edgbaston, and we had a long search before we settled for an old Victorian house on the South Circular Road, depressing for the children at first, but children adapt to anything with love and friends around them.

Two years after moving to Kew, I had our third baby, a boy, who arrived with great speed whilst colleagues at Queen Charlotte's Hospital were doing a research run on us both, monitoring foetal oxygen during labour. I had consented, being interested and a medic, but warned them that my labours were usually pretty brief and I might ruin the project – which I did. Baby appeared after a couple of contractions, protesting wildly about the wire attached to his head to monitor his oxygen levels, which was soon removed. I brought him home to meet his family, who were to move yet again to what became our family house and is still regarded as such. Keith's parents had died within 24 hours of each other during my pregnancy. His mother had cancer of unknown origin which overwhelmed her very quickly, and lovely Grandpa died of a heart attack the very next day, to be with his beloved Constance Mary. It was so moving and poignant. They were known to the children as Grandpa and Grandma Seaside because they lived in retirement from the RAF in Bognor Regis, that much joked-about resort. The modest amount of money they left us enabled us to move up the property field yet again, and we took the chance.

I had long coveted a large and mysterious old house behind a magnificent Ginkgo tree on Kew Gardens Road, which was owned by Professor Thomas, a retired professor from the Natural History Museum. She was also a member of the Liberal Party, of which I had been a member for some years, having joined in 1959 while at UCL, and I had collected her membership dues and delivered leaflets to her from time to time. She had died a few months before, and we jumped at the opportunity. We bought the house from her son, Jim Thomas, who still lives in Kew. It needed painting inside, and central heating had to be installed, but for our family, plus various friends, children and relatives who lived with us from time to time, it was heaven. Spacious and solid, with no frills, we partied and chased around that house until all the family had gone, and it was time once again to move on.

I love moving house – must be my traveller ancestry.

Chapter 6: Into Politics

At UCH, and later after qualifying, I became concerned that modern medicine was becoming too obsessed with individual diseases and their cure rather than prevention of disease in the first place. We could do more and more for fewer and fewer patients. I became interested in politics for that reason. It is no good treating the disease if we did nothing to improve the living conditions and lifestyles of our patients, which had led to the disease in the first place. I became a deliverer of leaflets and campaigner for the local Liberal candidate wherever our jobs took us. Political passion finally took hold after we moved to Kew, not long after another sudden death, that of my eldest brother, Michael, aged just forty years old, an accountant and administrator in public service who was planning to go into political life. My last conversation with him was about the choice he felt he had to make between Labour and our family's traditional leanings to the Liberals. He had had a myocardial infarction, a heart attack, three years earlier, and he and my sister-in-law Anne had confided in me that it could happen again. There were no stents or bypasses in those days. Three weeks bed rest and then home was the rule, and keep your fingers crossed! No crossing of fingers helped my brother, who had another infarct that killed him at the age of forty. Was there any escape from our family curse?

There is always a silver lining, though. Keith and I always regarded Michael's son and daughter as part of our family: Ted has had a great career in human resources and still makes us and his own family laugh, just as his father did. His sister Lizzie is my companion and tour guide on annual trips to the Edinburgh Festival. There seems to be nothing that she does not know about English literature and drama. I shall never know what my brother would have decided to do politically, but it made me even more determined to pick up his banner and carry on.

The seventies saw the birth and development of community politics promoted by a remarkable Kew Liberal councillor called Dr

Stanley Rundle. A similar exercise was going on in Liverpool under the tutelage of Sir Trevor Jones. Who started it is lost in the mists of time. The Liberals were certainly very active in Kew. Our family peace was disturbed one evening, just after we moved to Kew, by an earnest man, wearing, I remember, a longish dark blue mac, with a 'Save the Whale' badge on its lapel.

Dr Grant Lewison, who became a great friend and supporter, was on my doorstep to enrol me into the local party, having heard from a helper at my children's school that there was a very likely Liberal activist moved into the area. That person was Caroline Blomfield, and she and her husband, Liberal Councillor David Blomfield, were the inspirations of Kew Ward after Stanley Rundle sadly died of leukaemia.

Stanley and David taught me two valuable lessons in politics. Stanley always urged to tell the truth in politics because that way, the people would trust you, even when they didn't like what you said. He also added that it was useful if you had a bad memory because you would not have to remember which lie you had told! It sounds a bit simple and naive, but looking at the results of 'spin' as practised by all administrations subsequently, it was good advice. 'Spin' is political parlance for lies. David 'the Guru' Blomfield always stuck to principles and demonstrated to us all how important this is during a saga in Kew, which is engraved on my mind. The government of the day had decided to set up bail hostels for people awaiting trial who had nowhere to live. After long public consultation, Kew Liberals, who were in favour of the principle of bail hostels anyway, decided to promote and publicly support a hostel to be set up in Kew's old police station. This happened just before the 1978 local elections, and I was standing for the very first time in an election, alongside existing councillors David Blomfield and Leslie Worth. Our Conservative opponents ran a campaign against us, almost entirely on the bail hostel issue, even putting out a leaflet showing a man leaning out of a window dressed in prison clothes holding a dagger dripping blood. The caption was 'Kew Liberals gave you this'. It was so startling that even some of their own deliverers refused to distribute it. It was a baptism of fire for me. I could not believe that politicians could be so mean and dishonest, not just to us but to unconvicted men on bail—Tory justice for you. I failed to get in, and David and Leslie lost their seats.

David Blomfield, however, had no regrets: he proceeded to work even harder on issues in Kew and continued to support the new bail hostel. In less than a year, one Tory councillor had cut and run, and David gained a famous victory in the by-election that followed. Even more satisfying was when, two years later, another Tory lost his nerve and resigned, and I was elected councillor in Kew Ward with a huge majority. My first political victory. We never stopped supporting the bail hostel, which is still there and has brought no harm to Kew or its residents whatsoever. A famous victory for principle and my second lesson learned. Pompous though it may sound, I have always tried to tell the truth as I see it, and I always stick to those basic Liberal principles instilled in me by the Guru Blomfield and Dr Stanley Rundle. They have got me into some enormous scrapes and gained me many enemies, but no one in politics can please all of the people all of the time.

Local politics was easy enough to combine with family and medicine, thanks to the dear man I married. Being a local councillor means getting to know the people in your area well and finding out what bothers them. I am sad to say the issues that dominated were other people's planning applications (noise, dust and bother), other people's trees that shaded their garden (but never the tree in their garden which shaded their neighbour's) and dog mess on pavements. There were some really big housing problems and child care issues, but being a well-heeled area, these were not so frequent.

Before long, in 1981, the Liberals took control of the council, and I became Chair of Social Services. That was a different story. The problem of government cuts to local government loomed large, and that famous phrase 'efficiency savings' were bandied about by the Margaret Thatcher led Tory government. We could do little to improve the lot of children, the elderly and the mentally ill with the Tories in power. Homeless people piled up on the streets, and local people set up a centre where they could get meals and advice and raised funds for an overnight shelter and a bed for the night if they were at the top of the queue. The Vineyard Centre is still in Richmond, together with the night shelter on the roundabout. It is well used yet again as the next wave of homeless comes onto our streets, generated by Tory austerity policies.

I had the added problem of having to deal with a very difficult, and I thought not very competent, director of social services who cared little for his staff or the clients of the service but concentrated all his efforts on being a yes man to the chief executive. He was a bully too, and the staff were afraid of him, so they did not function at their best. It took me a year to persuade him to take early retirement. After that, the service ran more smoothly, and a new man was appointed, Richard Jeffries, who was loved by all and had done many jobs in social services from the bottom up after he left university. A rare find.

In May 1981, the Liberals won the Richmond seat on the Greater London Council by 815 votes, after Herculean efforts by the candidate Adrian Slade, one of the funniest and most charismatic people in the party. Whilst at Cambridge, he had been a founding member of the Footlights club from which emerged the iconic 'Beyond the Fringe' that had us all rolling in the aisles. At this time, Adrian was famous within the party for composing songs to be belted out with relish at party conferences accompanied by himself on the piano.

The result of the election was challenged by the Tories, whose main charge was that we had exceeded the number of garden stake posters erected during the campaign. Many of our supporters had made their own and had not cost us anything, but nevertheless, they took us to court. A full trial was held in the Council Chamber at York House in Twickenham, and I was a witness. This was my only experience of being involved in a court case, and at first could not take it seriously until I mounted the steps into the witness box and swore by Almighty God, to tell the truth, the whole truth, and nothing but the truth. An easy one for me because I always did.

After combing through the various sites where posters had been displayed, I was dismissed. After a week of this nonsense, the poor judge declared that we had overspent by sixpence but that each side should pay their own costs. In other words, he was saying a plague on us all. This was fine, of course, for the Conservatives, who had all the resources of Conservative Central Office behind them and many rich donors. For us Liberals, having spent out at the election, we were stuck, and to find in the region of £70,000 seemed an impossible task.

Adrian was undeterred. He contacted his old Cambridge Footlights friends, including John Cleese and the Pythons, the Goodies, Peter Cook, Rowan Atkinson and many other household names, and together with Adrian himself, his brother Julian of *Salad Days* fame, and other family members, they managed to secure Drury Lane for one night, and put together a wonderful show called *An Evening at Court,* which included a hilarious farce called *The Trial of Hadrian Slide*. The theatre that night was packed with Liberals and others, and we howled with laughter as the piss was thoroughly taken out of our opponents and the necessary money was raised.

Around this time, another great event took place for the Liberals on the national political scene. The 'Gang of Four', Shirley Williams, Bill Rogers, Roy Jenkins and David Owen, all big beasts in the Labour Party, had become sick of the left-wingers led by Michael Foot and had decided to defect and form a new party. It was hugely exciting at the time, and after a few abortive attempts at winning seats, the new Social Democratic Party formed an alliance with us Liberals, and it was thought, when opinion polls soared to great heights, that a new dawn was coming. It did not, of course. Despite all the excitement, we polled badly in 1987, and because of the first past the post electoral system, we gained only twenty-two seats in parliament. I am unable to give learned commentary on what went on during that time. I was back in the NHS full time, I had three children, was a local councillor and committee chair, so I had little spare time to find out what was going on. My most vivid memories are the rally at Llandudno that we all processed to one Saturday to witness the formation of the Alliance, I think. Standing at the back of the hall, I wept that day as Shirley Williams addressed us. I saw new hope for our future.

There followed a complicated but exhilarating time for the party, with our leader, David Steel, often battling with the arrogance of David Owen and being teased about it by the media. David Steel was a great leader. Calm, trusting of us and knowledgeable, without any of the pomposity displayed by many others. He was also capable of some rousing speeches to send us away from conferences, the most memorable being the one which sent us away with the exhortation: 'Go back to your constituencies and prepare for government.' We did, but of course, government was not within our grasp.

The other memory was Rosie Barnes' by-election in Greenwich in the early days of the SDP, which we were all commanded to attend. After a whole day of delivering tower blocks with our leaflets, I staggered back to base to say goodbye but was persuaded to deliver special letters to one more tower block on my way back to the station by the formidable Pat Wainwright, the Richmond agent, who had been sent to Greenwich to organise the campaign. I limped out and along the road to the last block of the day. Of course, the lift was broken, and I climbed ten or was it twelve flights of stairs, littered with rubbish and stinking of urine, delivering letters, individually addressed. Halfway back down, I found a letter I must have dropped, which was addressed to a resident on the top floor. I remembered a local election in Barnes where David Cornwell had won by *one* vote after several recounts, and that letter, I knew, in my crazed state, could be the one vote needed. Only people who have suffered from the electioneering bug will understand that, rather than ignore that one letter and carry on down, I climbed back up, reached the door of the flat where a big notice on top of their dustbin said, 'No more fucking election leaflets!'

I placed the letter carefully by the placard. Sad that it was my abiding memory of the SDP. Rosie Barnes did win the seat by more than one vote. Later, of course, with Shirley Williams and Adrian Slade in charge, a new party, the Social and Liberal Democrats, came into being, much to the disgust of David Owen, who remained outside. The LibDems were born. Why Adrian Slade was not given a peerage at that time, I shall never fathom. I heard it said that he had 'given too much away to the SDP', but I have no idea what that meant. The shenanigans of party hierarchies, I suppose, but we could do with him in the House of Lords.

I had at that time just gone back to the NHS as a full-time doctor, responsible for Women's Services in Ealing Health Authority based in Southall, Middlesex, a good half an hour away from home by car. The job was a wonderful opportunity to improve services for women by liaising with GPs and expanding services for women in particular. As well as family planning clinics, a new breast screening service had to be set up, and women had to be encouraged to come along for the newly created cervical cytology tests too. Southall was particularly interesting because we had a huge Asian population there, later joined by Somalis, Afghans, and the already existing large Polish enclave at the Acton end of Ealing. Persuading women to have smear tests and talk about family planning often included contacting community leaders. My chief nursing officer was a bundle of energy called Doreen Burchett, who was happy to talk to gurus and imams. She came back triumphant one day, having persuaded an imam that smear tests were a good thing and he should encourage the women in his flock to come along for a test. He did so on the condition that the clinic was set up in the mosque so that he could supervise! Only in an administrative sense, of course, but it added to our problems of keeping all services confidential. The young women were controlled by the older women, but the men were in charge always.

Education was probably more important than anything else in the eighties in Southall, and Featherstone High School was, and still is, a very successful school. It did not prevent old traditions prevailing, though. I remember, in particular, twin girls who had done extremely well in their A Levels and came from a loving family. They asked me for family planning advice because they were travelling out to India to be married. They would have liked to go on to further education but did not want to let their parents down. So sad and such a waste. Arranged, forced, and child marriages were all much too common in those days and led to the foundation of the brave 'Black Sisters of Southall', who were one of the first groups to start campaigning for women's rights and providing help to girls caught in family traps.

Another girl I had seen and confirmed her early, accidental pregnancy was very distressed and did not know what would happen to her. Extensive enquiries about her led to a dead end. Nobody knew where she had gone or what had happened. Abortion had been legal since 1968 thanks to David Steel's 1967 Act, but it still required visits to two doctors and the inevitable loss of privacy in a society that was so closely knit. I dreaded to think of what happened to that girl and remembered as a junior doctor before the act, the ghastly cases I had seen when women died as a result of illegal back street abortions.

On another occasion, a Somali girl and university graduate came into one of my clinics and asked to have a smear test which was my first encounter with female genital mutilation, which I was to tackle much later on in parliament. She was referred to our gynaecologists, and we all began to realise what a problem it was for the midwives and obstetricians responsible for the safe delivery of babies and understanding what women wanted afterwards. Some wanted to be sewn up as they were before, and it was not until we got some good interpreters that we could really tackle the problem. I have nothing but admiration for these refugee women who often escape with their children, probably never to see their men again, into an alien world that does not understand their culture.

In the same year, I was alerted by social workers in the area that they had found accommodation for a mother and three children in a room near the clinic, but she needed medical attention. None of the local GPs would make a home visit, so I went along with an interpreter as the only medic around. I found a dingy room with one mattress and a fridge – both luxuries provided by social services. On the mattress lay a very sick woman being crawled over by some very frightened toddlers and a baby. That woman was the wife of a doctor in Mogadishu, Somalia, who had been bundled onto a plane by her husband as the enemy approached. She had run out of medicine and had an open tubercular abscess in her neck, which was in a dreadful mess. After ordering the appropriate treatment and getting the local people to help her, we gradually resolved the situation. I often wondered how I would have coped in that situation if I was caught in a bloody civil war. So many tragedies, but nothing to what I would experience in the field of international development when I went into parliament.

Something else which I would experience in parliament one day was introduced to me by a consultant in public health in Ealing, with whom I became friendly. She was Dr Ghada Karmi. Talking to her one lunchtime, I was saying how unhappy with the health service my team of mostly Asian women doctors were. She laughingly responded that if they were not happy, they should go home – they *had* a home to go to. Ghada then explained that she was Palestinian and all of her family had been expelled from their home during the 'Nakba', the 'catastrophe' for Palestinians, driven from their land when the state of Israel was created. I learned a lot that lunchtime, which was to transform my view of the Holy Land and shape my political career in the most amazing way when I eventually got to Westminster.

My life then was a juggling session between school runs, council duties in Twickenham, and the health service. All were dear to my heart, and I had to have an au pair from Switzerland to help me juggle. She was the first of three lovely girls, all child-loving and all determined to learn English. They all enhanced our family. They were like much older sisters to the children and took them swimming and walking if there was a time when I couldn't. I even managed to teach the first one, Clare Muller, to drive, and she passed her test! We were thrilled. They were succeeded by a nurse in between training who was equally lovable and had a boyfriend who joined her some evenings when he had finished work. Those busy years in my parallel careers of medicine and politics were helped and enhanced by those young women.

One brilliant opportunity to travel was offered to me by a local Labour Party supporter/trade unionist who nevertheless supported the LibDems in national elections. He was getting together a medical delegation to go to East Germany to see medical facilities there and experience real 'socialism' in action. Before that trip, I had not thought that for the ordinary citizen, life would be very much different from life here if you stayed out of politics and kept your head down. How wrong I was.

The first experience was at Check Point Charlie, which we had to cross to get into East Berlin. We were fed one by one with our luggage into a tight little corridor, and the door slammed shut after each one. I dragged my case in behind me and stood to attention as the official behind the screen beside me scrutinised my passport. Just as he was about to hand it back to me, there was a loud ringing sound which I quickly realised was coming from my suitcase. I grabbed it and tried to open it in the confined space. I rummaged away as the official face of East Germany got redder and redder. Eventually, I delivered my alarm clock merrily ringing and held it aloft for inspection. I wish I could say it raised a smile, but it did not, just a scowl and a click as he released the door at the other end of the space and waved me on. I fell out giggling to concerned colleagues looking on. They had worried about me! I asked one of them what the German for 'apologies' was and learned the word 'entschuldigung', which I shouted back to the guards. Our German guide was very amused and said that the English go round the world, saying sorry. Apparently, we are famous for it.

Life in East Berlin was tough. Everything your heart could desire was on display in the 'duty-free' shops but could only be purchased with West German marks, so they were out of reach for most East Germans. We had a government minder with us for the whole trip, and during a moment in the middle of a park where we had gone for fresh air, my interpreter told me that they were listening in to everything and all closed spaces were bugged. We could only speak relatively freely in the open air away from buildings. Food, whilst we were there, had cream on everything, sweet or savoury. It was explained that they had a glut of dairy produce that had to be eaten, like it or not. On the other hand, there was very little fruit or vegetables anywhere. East Germans ate what they were given. There were no homeless people, and everyone had some sort of job.

The Professor of Paediatrics we met at the very good children's hospital there invited us back to his two-bedroom flat for tea. He had the same accommodation as any worker in East Germany, suited roughly to his family size. All men were equal? All women were too and seemed to have equal status, in the professions at least. East Berlin was a lesson learned and doubled my delight when the wall came down on that glorious day in November 1989. My interpreter there sent me a little piece of it as a souvenir. I still weep when I hear the Choral Symphony and the Song for Europe, just as I did that night we watched television as it was played in East Berlin in those early days. It fuelled my passion for the European Union.

I experienced another culture accompanying Keith on a lecture tour he gave in Japan, where he had made links with radiologists wanting to train in the UK. Japan was even stranger than East Germany but is now a common tourist destination. When we were there, I was treated as a token man because women, particularly after marriage, did not go out with their husbands or entertain guests at home. If they had trained professionally, they did not work after marriage: the home and children were their whole world. In the last few decades, Japanese women have liberated themselves and have more freedom, thank goodness. We were lucky to live in Kew because Japanese businessmen came over with their families and rented houses near us, so the children had Japanese friends at school, and we were able to see them when we visited and penetrate the 'private' lives of Japanese families.

During these early adventures, my mother came to supplement the care being given by our girls, and everyone was happy to be spoiled. She was by now in her late seventies and decided to move to Kew. She lived in a flat just around the corner from us, only half of which she could afford from the sale of her three-bedroomed house in the Midlands, an illustration of the great divide between the affluent southeast and the rest of the country. We took out an extra mortgage to fund the other half of her flat, being more prosperous by then. Keith had secured a post as consultant neuroradiologist at St Thomas' Hospital, and we were financially secure for the first time in our lives together.

I consider myself to be quite hardworking, but I honestly could not have done what I did without the help of these other women. Men have a permanent housekeeper, cook and childminder, and whatever the 'modern' husband does in the home, in most homes, it is the female partner who shoulders the main burden. Will it ever change? I doubt it. Men will help more and more, but whilst women have a uterus and breasts and oestrogen pumping around their bodies for a good part of our adult life, they will remain the carers. The great advantage it gives us women is the variety we have in our lives if we play the game well, and of course, are lucky enough to get an education. Pity the poor male who has to carry on working until retirement with few opportunities for a break. However, it did not stop me wondering how I would have fared with my skills as a man with a wife and family, not the other way round. Discuss, as they say in exam papers.

Chapter 7: Honourable Member

The parliamentary seat became vacant in Richmond after Alan Watson, who had tried and failed to win for the LibDems, decided to give way for another candidate, and I was selected for the seat of Richmond and Barnes to fight the 1992 General Election.

My mother, who had supported everything I did in my life, died just after I was selected. She would have preferred me to stick to medicine. She saw politics as a dirty business, although she always voted. For her, it was an obligation for women, hard-won when she was a schoolgirl. It was so sad she did not live to see the fun. One of the saddest things for me was that just after she died, I was invited, as a prominent prospective parliamentary candidate for the LibDems, to take part in Any Questions on Radio 4. Since my father died years before, my mother had Radio 4 on constantly, day and night. She knew the time of day by it, she knew all the personalities and programmes, and she was steeped in current affairs. She was not afraid of expressing her opinions either, which were always worth listening to, based as they were on her life experiences of two world wars and a teaching career. Radio 4 was my mother's constant companion, and her favourite programme of all was Any Questions. My ancient Aunt Floss, my mother's eldest sister, rang me the next day to tell me how, through tears of pride and joy, she had turned the radio up very loud so that my mother could hear it 'up there'!

That was the election we thought we had in the bag at last, after three near misses by Alan Watson, who now sits as a Liberal Democrat in the House of Lords. The 1992 campaign was great fun. We were in the eye of the media as the LibDems' most winnable seat. Paddy Ashdown made several visits and strode about at a great pace with me staggering behind, trying to keep up on smart high heels. He is an exhausting man to work with – his wife should have had the knighthood for valour! This was the election when Des Wilson, our Campaign Manager, insisted on all candidates, women and men, being advised on their appearance, including the wearing of high heels, causing me to spend a fortune on clothes to enhance my 'soft autumn' colouring. This was the election when Keith Tonge's old yellow, ex-army Land Rover rumbled all over the constituency in the days CO_2 emissions became an issue. It was driven by a friend of my eldest son, David, who also came out with us as the campaign photographer. The same Land Rover ferried Paddy around on his visits and was once famously pushed back physically by the sitting Conservative MP, Jeremy Hanley, in the hope a camera would catch him doing it when he would declare that he was resisting the tide of Liberalism. He was such a good-natured man.

This was also the election when a break-in at Paddy Ashdown's lawyer's office had revealed evidence of an affair between Paddy and a secretary years before. What sort of news was that? What man hasn't? I have a French friend who cannot understand the English attitude to the odd extramarital affair. 'In France, you do not think your man is worth 'aving unless someone else wants 'im,' was her comment. The Sun newspaper, however, smelling blood, came up with the brilliant headline 'Paddy Pants Down'. This was dealt with by total honesty from Paddy.

The night before the news broke, he made a personal phone call to all his candidates in key seats up and down the country. We all respected him even more, and his personal ratings soared in the polls. The only comment I received on the doorstep was from an old lady in Mortlake who told me she had sent off a Tory canvasser who had been saying how dreadful it all was, with the famous remark, 'I told her. I wish that nice Mr Ashdown would come round here and do to me what he did to her. He's lovely, their leader.' Most of us candidates agreed. He was inspirational if sometimes wrong and would always listen to contrary arguments and stay on good terms with whoever challenged him.

The legend goes that a commanding officer once asked to give a reference for Paddy said of him, 'His men will follow him anywhere – out of sheer curiosity.' We knew what that officer meant, and long after he stood down as leader, he was still a shining personality in the party. His death in 2019 was a cruel blow, after several years enlivening the House of Lords.

That election in 1992 was one we thought we had in the bag until the last week, when Neil Kinnock, after a glitzy final rally in Sheffield, scared off all the punters who thought he could not possibly be the next Prime Minister and they all voted Conservative, for safety – and John Major! All our lovely Labour tactical voters, all those Tory swingers, all came to nothing, and I lost. My one abiding memory is sitting in The Sun Inn in Richmond after the count (specially open for us), feeling sad but relieved it was all over and comforting my weeping daughter, who had kept the home fires burning for me during the campaign as well as doing her share of delivering and getting her friends on board to do the same. She wept for the entire party!

During that election, Torkild Strandberg, a young lawyer from the Swedish Liberal party, came over to help and was enamoured with our electioneering methods. He invited me over to his town, Landskrona, near Malmö, to talk to the activists in his party there. The winter was so cold that the normal ferry from Copenhagen had been replaced by an icebreaker with no food or hot drinks on board. It took a long and freezing time to get across the Skagerrak Strait. After a freezing 24 hours giving talks to party activists, we went over to Helsingør (Hamlet's Elsinore) in Denmark to stand on the battlements of the castle and recite Shakespeare, but it was so cold we beat a hasty retreat back to Landskrona and hot chocolate.

Despite such adventures, I remained deflated and a little depressed after that election. Funny though, election campaigns are a bit like childbirth. The exhaustion and pain at the end make you vow you will never do it again, but the memory fades quickly, and two years later, I found myself at the hustings in the newly named and boundary-changed constituency of Richmond Park that incorporated North Kingston, winning the selection process again against opponents Chris Fox, who gave up active politics but now sits in the House of Lords, and one Mark Oaten who became Liberal Democrat MP for Winchester. Both men, I remember thinking at the time, were much better candidates than me. Let history be our judge. I went on to win the seat, the first non-Conservative and the first woman to represent the area.

Liberals and LibDems had a favourite song which we sang on 'glee club' night at party conferences year after year. It went something like,

> 'The people's flag is slightly pink,
> It's not so red as you may think.'

Neil Kinnock, and Tony Blair after him, had transformed the Labour Party into an electable and very fresh new party that swept to power in 1997. The Liberal Democrats benefitted because to keep the Tories out, Labour voters were persuaded to vote for us. We convinced people that a Labour vote was a wasted vote in some Tory constituencies. So it was. I won Richmond Park with the help of Labour voters who I never forgot to thank. I had a brilliant organizer, Louise Arimatsu, who, even before we had an office to work from, turned her bedroom upside down, and we sat on the edge of her bed, side by side, concocting articles for the press and reviewing leaflets. She had a computer – I did not!

My youngest son was in his gap year and had volunteered to help. He took over a whole derelict ward and ensured that we won it, under the guidance of Louise, David Williams, my agent and leader of the council in Richmond, John Tilley, LibDem leader in Kingston, and Peter Grender, the Chairman of Kingston LibDems. He also came into my office for a while after the election as a volunteer, and I like to think that my interest in international development led to him becoming a geologist and engineer. Perhaps not. The overall Chairman of my campaign was Adrian Slade. David Williams was an old warhorse of elections and tactics. His knowledge of previous elections used to enthral or bore people depending on your taste. Anyway, he knew the lot. On one training weekend for candidates in key seats, we were subjected to a very light-hearted political quiz at dinner one evening by Chris Rennard, the party's election guru. Our table was struggling until I, as captain, asked if anyone had a mobile phone. They did. We spent the rest of the quiz on it, writing down the answers given to us by David Williams on the other end of the line. We won, but after a well-justified and good-natured complaint from the other teams, we were disqualified and lost the bottle of champagne. We were commended on our initiative and enterprise and given a bottle anyway! With the help of these people and an amazing team, the election campaign progressed.

The electorate was thoroughly fed up with the Conservatives. Labour, led by Tony Blair, won a landslide, with Liberal Democrats picking up a swathe of seats up and down the country, including Richmond Park. It felt like a new dawn. I was a member of the House of Commons, and two days later, I was giving out the prizes for the cat show at Richmond May Fair. You can't climb much higher than that! Someone remarked that they had not felt so happy since the end of the Second World War, which seemed a bit over the top for a slightly apprehensive me, wondering what Westminster would be like.

Two days later, I entered the Palace of Westminster. I had never been inside before, although I had stood outside as a child with my parents, listening to Big Ben. No, I never stood on the steps of 10 Downing Street, like more precocious children have done. I knew my place. A little girl in the fifties would not dream of doing that! My adventures had begun, and I was in constant demand during those first few weeks, as were many of us, to describe what it was like being an MP. In the first week, I was on Woman's Hour on Radio 4 with Virginia Bottomley, who was waxing eloquently about the place and how wonderful it was. I just didn't see it like that in the early days. It was fake Gothic, rambling and difficult to navigate one's way around.

The Palace of Westminster is like a huge, ancient university or public school, but I wouldn't know because I went to a state grammar school and UCL. More recently, it's been described as Hogwarts, but I wouldn't know about that either because I am not a Harry Potter fan – much too scary. It's certainly, dark, spooky, Victorian Gothic at its most magnificent, but in the back of my mind lurked irreverent thoughts about Disney and theme parks, perhaps Dracula's castle, or that castle we visited on our honeymoon, Neuschwanstein in Bavaria, built by Mad King Ludwig. I exclude from those remarks the greatest indoor space in England, namely Westminster Hall, the original site of English law and democracy, the setting for hideous trials followed by even more hideous hangings, drawings and quarterings up in Whitehall. The largest hammer-beam roof in Europe could tell some tales. In my darkest moments over the last ten years, I have made my way down to Westminster Hall to sit and think, and thank whoever is in charge up there, if anyone is, for my minor difficulties, compared with the brave souls who suffered here in the course of British history. One day I took a party of Palestinian teenagers from Abu Dis, near Jerusalem, into Westminster Hall and, after looking rather bored at first, they thrilled to the tale of Braveheart, being condemned to death in that very place. Even they had heard of Braveheart, thanks to Mel Gibson.

The first few days were a bit like changing schools. You know, when everyone seems to know where to go except you and everyone has friends except you. The truth is, of course, that nobody knows except the 'old boys', and they are determined not to help anyone because they had to find out by trial and error. The greatest offenders were my party, and the fact that we had only three women in the parliamentary party did not help. I will not name names, but we were purposefully ignored by a few. The first problem is the rabbit holes. There are great long corridors at Westminster, but many doors off them lead down staircases to I know not where, just like rabbit holes. I once found myself in an open space surrounded by high walls and half-filled with builders' rubble and equipment. I had to haul myself back up the stairs to a corridor and ask a passing policeman for help! Eventually, you work out a set of rabbit holes for yourself and learn to get about, but I have never met anyone who has not got lost or still gets lost on occasions. Who will be first with an App for the Palace of Westminster? It will never happen now because security is so tight, and no one must know their way around.

The next challenge is parliamentary procedure, which you just have to pick up as you go along. When to stand up, when to sit down, how to address one's colleagues (never directly, only through the Speaker). It goes on and on, and I found it completely hilarious. It was even necessary then to find the top hat at the end of your bench and place it on your head before making a point of order. That was dispensed with quickly by the new caring, sharing, snap crackle and pop Blair government, so I never got to wear it. A pity that! I have chided myself endlessly ever since for missing that opportunity. The men seem to get terribly fussed about people making mistakes and were great sticklers for procedure and taking you on one side to 'put you right' in the tea room. Thank you to all the MPs in the House who take a more relaxed view. I suppose if you are seen to know the rules, behave impeccably and never upset your colleagues or the party membership, you are more likely to be made a prefect or progress up the greasy pole of a political career. They also become boring and untrustworthy. It becomes obvious early on who the real politicians are and who is there because they feel passionately about issues. I met a wonderful African politician on my travels who said it was the same the whole world over, and always to remember that politicians are like monkeys – the higher they climb up the coconut tree, the more you can see of their backsides.

The House of Commons in 1997 was an impressive sight. I remember sitting on the LibDem benches, at my first Prime Minister's Question Time, when the House was packed, and thinking what a great spectacle it was. Still too few women and ethnic minorities, but the Labour Party's all-women shortlists had brought many more in. Bernie Grant, in his tribal robes, was worth a few glances. David Blunkett and his guide dog looking terribly bored, and Anne Begg in her wheelchair added more interest. The fact that all sorts and conditions of men and women were there, from manual workers to professors, gave the place a more representative air. Prime Minister's Questions is the event of the week and has nothing to do with politics or policy. It is pure theatre with some actors better than others. It is a verbal duel watched all over the world and to be in the crowd is fun, pure fun. It's like a rugby crowd before too much beer has been drunk (although a fair amount *will* have been drunk by this crowd too). The jokes and asides and general goings-on are just great and make up for all the arrogance displayed by a lot of MPs the rest of the time.

Some of the women, sadly, were offended by remarks made, and one even asked me to go with her to the Speaker to complain about the 'rude' gestures made by a certain extremely confident Tory who always had a good lunch. As a graduate of medical school in the early sixties, when there were few women in our year, I had been brought up on male rudeness, so I declined but sympathised. Perhaps I had developed a fairly thick hide to shake off such insults. I think I was wrong not to take it more seriously. I have sympathy for women who have to tolerate the sexual antics of men in power but give as good as you get was my mother's dictum and *never* lose your sense of humour.

The way to deal with rude gestures is to beat them at their own game. One LibDem MP thought it was great fun to place his hand on the bit of bench you were about to occupy so that with luck, you would leap up in horror. After a couple of times suffering his bit of fun, I returned the compliment one day, and as he sat down beside me, I placed my hand, fingers in a claw shape, to catch him as he sat down. His face was a picture. We remain the best of friends. It is a very different position if the man doing the harassment is in some position of power over you, and in recent years more and more cases have come to light showing that in some industries, particularly the film industry, the only way to get ahead is to allow sexual harassment and often sleep with the 'boss'. It is disgusting and just as well that many women are ignoring tough old birds like me and making it public. Jobs and advancing your career should not depend on giving sexual favours. It should be reported and quickly. I can honestly say that nothing has ever happened to me that I was not able to cope with immediately. Maybe I am not that attractive? Answers on a postcard, please.

A great haven, and the place really to do some work, is the members' library. I was directed there when, in the week after the General Election, I desperately needed to have a quick power nap before being required to do the BBC's Question Time in the evening. My office was too busy and noisy, so I asked a doorkeeper where I could go. 'They all sleep in the library, ma'am,' I was told. It was true. There they all were up at the far end of the magnificent place, away from the tables and computers, slumbering and snoring away in two rows of armchairs facing each other. I had an overwhelming urge to pop a dummy in the mouths of the more restless ones, but instead settled down, feet on a footstool, and had a very refreshing half an hour. I am an expert power napper, having learned the art when I was a junior hospital doctor whilst waiting for the next patient to be admitted.

In those early months, I tried to introduce an issue that I had felt strongly about as a Women's Health manager and doctor in the NHS. In my first week, I made an appointment to see the Secretary of State for Health, Frank Dobson. It had always seemed to be an insult to women that they had to see a doctor for emergency contraception, commonly known as the 'Morning After Pill'. It was, and is, a very safe and effective method of prevention of pregnancy for a woman who has forgotten her pills or got carried away and took a risk. Frank Dobson and his Minister, the extremely impressive Yvette Cooper, were enthusiastic, and the wheels were set in motion to prepare the ground in association with Schering Pharmaceuticals, who were producing a properly packaged version of Post Coital Contraception or PCC as it is known in the trade.

Vanessa Haines, my Parliamentary researcher, a clever and enthusiastic ally, set to work on a campaign which we waged over the next year or so. *Cosmopolitan* magazine was enthused and wrote a whole two-page spread on the subject. A press conference was held in Westminster to tell the world that the new pill would be available over the counter, without seeing a doctor, and would be free in Family Planning Clinics or local surgeries. We were not without our critics, of course: the Daily Express – it had to be – splashed the headlines 'MP calls for abortion over the counter', encouraging what I came to call the 'zealots' to bombard me with letters and phone calls, some very abusive, but I was used to that having worked to set up good abortion services in my health authority. Working in the field of reproductive and sexual health for many years had got me used to campaigners against abortion and birth control. Some people seem to think they can impose their strongly held views on everyone else. I have always defended a woman's right to choose and frankly think it is no one else's business. If the zealots think it is a sin, then they do not have to do it themselves. Nevertheless, it happened. The morning after pill became freely available and is one of my proudest achievements.

Paddy Ashdown had first asked me to be in the Treasury team with Malcolm Bruce. A great shock this was but had resulted from my interest in hypothecated taxes, especially for the NHS. Paddy saw an opportunity for me to practice what I had preached. Fortunately, I had Louise Arimatsu, my organiser from the election victory, by my side. She had opted to be my researcher for the first few months at Westminster until we were all bedded down. Louise is Anglo-Japanese and quite brilliant at everything she does. After a couple of degrees, one in Tokyo and one in London, she worked for Nomura Investments. She had 'retired' a few years later with a small private income to help the LibDems! I was the lucky LibDem who benefited from Louise. Just as we were becoming used to the idea of me as a Treasury spokesman, I was walking across a car park in Richmond on my way to a meeting when my shiny new mobile phone rang – funny to think they were relatively 'new' in 1998. It was Paddy in assertive mode.

'Jenny, is this phone secure?'

'Er – I suppose so. I'm in a car park.'

'I need to take you off the Treasury team.'

'Oh. Right. Why is that?' (trying to mask the relief in my voice.)

'I put Vince Cable into International Development, but he has told me he cannot do it because he used to work for Shell, and the NGOs will persecute him.' (Shell had been much criticised for unethical behaviour in Nigeria.)

'Oh, that means I can be on the backbenches? I know the health brief has been filled.'

'No, I like the idea of you taking on Clare Short in International Development. I want you to do that.' The phone went dead. I saluted smartly and continue on my way to my meeting, imagining Paddy watching Clare and me wrestle in the mud somewhere on the Dark Continent. Lovely man!

The Daily Mail contacted me soon after the election and my elevation to the shadow ministries of state. They wanted an interview and suggested a restaurant in Soho at lunchtime the next day. Not a happy experience. I spent nearly an hour waiting for this chap at the bar of a rather sleazy place, sipping lime and soda and receiving very odd glances from fellow diners and passers-by. When I eventually managed to contact my Daily Mail man, I discovered that I had been waiting in one of Soho's 'knocking shops', no doubt treated with tact by the locals, as a poor old girl long passed her prime, but down on her luck and trying to earn a few bob in the lunchtime. The subsequent article in the newspaper was enlivened by this experience. I thank my lucky stars. I wasn't forcibly removed by some pimp protecting his territory. I guess they decided there was no competition. My self-worth received another blow a few months later when rushing down Victoria Street from one meeting to another at Westminster. I was stopped by an old tramp who wagged his finger at me and said, 'Gerroff the streets, you old trollop'. But I digress.

Chapter 8: International Development

Many people have asked, and indeed I have asked myself, why, after over thirty years in the NHS, with wide experience in clinical and management work, married to a consultant in a teaching hospital, with the added experience of chairing the party's health policy panel and heading up a group looking at hypothecation of taxes for the NHS – why, after all that, the party leader rejected that knowledge and expertise, giving the health job to one of his cronies. Buggins' turn, I guess. Men are like that, and nowhere are they more like that than in politics. I decided to knuckle down and learn a new subject. I was helped by Keith, who came home the following day with an atlas because he knew I would need it, having given up geography to concentrate on sciences at school.

Soon after being made spokesperson/man/woman for International Development, I received an invitation to the Locarno Rooms of the Foreign and Commonwealth Office (FCO) to hear Robin Cook, Foreign Secretary, deliver his first major speech. The Locarno Rooms are Whitehall's best-kept secret. They had been divided into separate little rooms in the fifties for various civil servants' offices and filled with filing cabinets and neon strip lighting. Mrs Thatcher realised what was there and insisted on their restoration. The Foreign Office itself is awe-inspiring with its brilliant courtyard and staircase leading up to the main rooms. This staircase is painted with scenes of 'humble' delegates from the colonies bearing gifts and moving up towards the Great British Empress, Victoria. Even Washington has nothing quite as intimidating. The Locarno Rooms are just as grand and even more beautiful. Sadly, the FCO only has one or two open days a year, and visitors have to book in advance and nowadays run the gauntlet of security checks. Durbar Court, an inner courtyard in the India Office, is also stunning. Thank you, Mrs Thatcher, for all of that anyway.

I duly attended the FCO to hear Robin Cook's great speech. This was when he talked of a foreign policy with an ethical dimension – not an ethical foreign policy – there is a difference. He also talked of arms control and new legislation to be introduced, following his brilliant exposé of the Conservative government following the Scott report. He spoke of upholding Human Rights consistently, not just for our national interest. He pledged to make the UK a force for good in the world. 'Oh, brave new world that has such creatures in it,' I quoted to myself, as the goosebumps rose with excitement and emotion. It was not just me either. Plenty of civil servants and MPs looked pretty wet-eyed that afternoon. What a falling-off was there, as Robin Cook, the honest politician, gradually realised that his vision was not shared by his leader, except for window-dressing purposes. Robin's early death in 2005, at the age of only 59, was a huge loss to this country. Nevertheless, those early days were so filled with the hope of a new world order.

My first trip abroad brought me back to earth. I was sent to Warsaw for the parliamentary assembly of the Organisation for Security and Cooperation in Europe (OSCE). It was an introduction to the so-called 'jollies' enjoyed by MPs. We were treated to business class travel and a splendid five-star hotel in Warsaw near the restored Old City. I am not sure exactly what these assemblies are supposed to do. We passed resolutions which went nowhere – in fact, at the second such assembly I went to, the following year in Copenhagen, I asked what progress had been made on the resolutions from Warsaw, but answer came there none. In fact, the secretariat seemed a little shocked that anyone should have posed the question! The only value I can see is that they do forge links between parliamentarians from different countries – the OSCE includes the USA and Russia, so it was considered to be valuable just for that. There are so many for parliamentarians, as well as the actual officials of the organisations who meet relentlessly. The OSCE, OECD (the Organisation for Economic Co-operation and Development), NATO (the North Atlantic Treaty Organisation), parliamentary assemblies, the Council of Europe and many others all provide opportunities for parliamentarians to eat and drink together!

A memorable meeting was in Cairo, where European countries had been encouraged to send women parliamentarians to meet with our sister MPs from the Arab States. It was fascinating to compare different lives and freedoms, and we were given a good experience of Egypt. An obligatory trip to the Great Pyramid and the Sphinx in the very early morning to avoid the hawkers was just magical. We arrived at dawn with the site deserted and climbed up through the inside of the great pyramid to the King's Chamber, which was good exercise, although one or two women decided to give it a miss. When we emerged blinking into the morning sunshine, the camels had arrived with hundreds of hawkers to persuade us to buy necklaces, lucky charms and plaster models of dogs and cats, and, of course, King Tut. The final evening was spent at a musical evening at the Merchant's House in Old Cairo, the former home of Naguib Mahfouz, the great Egyptian writer, author of the *Cairo Trilogy*. Lit by oil lamps, we wandered the rooms and imagined being in purdah, looking down on the entertainment from the grilled windows of the women's rooms. It is a situation that still applies to many women all over the world. It was good to be reminded of the privileges we have won for ourselves in the west and the rights we now have.

That first summer recess was busy. My team and I had been running the constituency office from our study at home, in Kew. Luckily our family house in my constituency was a big old Victorian place that had comfortably swallowed our three children as well as assorted friends and relatives who lived with us from time to time. It was famous for Keith and me being able to sit in the sitting room with a glass of wine and the newspaper on a Saturday evening and not be able to hear the teenage party raging on the floors above. They don't make houses like that anymore! Acting as the constituency office was just another task that was required of our house whilst we searched Richmond for an affordable pad for the new Liberal Democrat MP and her staff. We held surgeries there every week too. My rock at that time, my head of office and a local councillor to boot was Nick Carthew, son of Alison Cornish, another local councillor, who had become a great friend and advisor during my early years in Richmond.

Chapter 9: Montserrat

My first foray as International Development Spokesman came when the Soufrière Hills Volcano in the Caribbean island of Montserrat started erupting again. It had done so several times over the past year, but the previous government had not given much attention to the Montserratians, who were, after all, citizens of one of Britain's Overseas Territories and as such should have been given maximum help in relocation until the eruptions stopped. I walked into our Whips' Office one morning and was told there was to be a statement on Montserrat in the House of Commons, and I had to 'take it'. That meant I had to get in there and ask the formidable Clare Short a question. My immediate reaction was, 'Where's Montserrat?' Having given up geography before O Levels, the only one I could think of was the one near Barcelona, which I had recently visited on holiday. I soon found out a huge amount about Montserrat, and the sufferings of the islanders were to play a huge part in my introduction to International Development over many weeks that followed.

Despite constituency business which was pouring in, the escalating crisis in Montserrat could not be avoided. The volcano was getting more and more active, and people had been killed trying to salvage possessions from their properties overcome by pyroclastic flows, a new term to me with which I was to become very familiar. It is what killed most people in Pompeii – hot toxic gases pouring down the mountainside in advance of the lava and engulfing everything. Questions were being asked about Britain's responsibility for the Montserratians who were being shunned by Antigua as they flooded in and treated very poorly if they came to the UK, certainly not as British citizens from one of our Dependent Territories. In those days, they had no right to come to the UK and no entitlements. In fact, those refugees from the volcano struggled to get any help at all in the first two years, before a wonderful woman called Janice Panton, a native of Montserrat who had been working as a legal secretary in the city, decided to set up a helpline and advice centre to steer the refugees through the housing and welfare systems in the UK. She was encouraged by her ex-boss Sally Hamwee, a friend of mine from Richmond Council days, who had been elevated to the House of Lords by Paddy Ashdown a few years before. Janice was brilliant and is now Janice Panton MBE. For the record, she now heads the Government of Montserrat Office in the UK and is her people's representative.

I had asked many questions about the situation before the recess and received assurances that everything possible was being done, the usual patter from government ministers. On one occasion, I had asked about the predictions of the experts and had become totally lost for the right word to describe a scientist who knows about volcanoes. Labour wags opposite me in the chamber had flapped their ears and pointed to John Redwood, the Tory MP known for his alien ways and popularly known as the 'Vulcan', like Mr Spock in Star Trek. Anyway, it worked, and I spat out 'vulcanologist' just in time to stop the Speaker from intervening in the joke. Funny, it was *not* for the people of Montserrat, who had been enjoying a tropical and affluent lifestyle with plenty of rich tourists to fill the island's coffers before disaster struck.

I decided, new MP or not, that the recently created Select Committee for International Development, of which I was a member, ought to become involved. I contacted our Chairman, Tory MP Bowen Wells, the nicest Conservative at Westminster, with a wealth of development experience in the Commonwealth Development Corporation and international trade. In less than a week, we were on our way to the Caribbean. Our party consisted of Bernie Grant, Labour MP for Haringey and well-known in the Caribbean, Ann Clwyd, Labour MP and Chair of the Human Rights All-Party Group, Dennis Canavan, fiercely Old Labour and Scots, Bowen Wells and myself, with the committee clerk to shepherd us. My first overseas adventure had begun. On arrival at Antigua Airport, we were mobbed by crowds, all personal friends of Bernie. Or at least he behaved as if they were. Smiling and waving from his buggy – he couldn't walk very far because of diabetic complications in the arteries of his legs – he sailed through the airport accompanied by cheers, followed by us mere mortals trotting obediently behind with our suitcases. A nice reversal of colonial times, I thought!

Our hotel was full of British holidaymakers who had not seen the sun for the whole of their holiday, blotted out as it was by clouds of volcanic ash blown over from Montserrat. They sat on the beach day after day in the gloom and could not even go and see the source of their misery which was out of bounds. The volcano was obvious enough, even from Antigua. A couple of times a day, there would be a greater or lesser explosion, and a mushroom cloud would rise over the island, just across the strait, where we were to go the next day by a government helicopter. The next morning, sure enough, we were loaded into a helicopter, earmuffs in place, and flew through the dust and gloom to the volcano island. I was beginning to feel like *Five go on an Adventure*, those books that used to terrify me – yes, even Enid Blyton could terrify me when I was a child.

It's funny how trusting you can be of the people charged with your welfare. Luckily I have always been like that. If I cannot *do* anything to improve safety because of a lack of knowledge or strength, I just relax! There are always exceptions, and I could not shut up when in the passenger seat of a car my husband was driving, but then he drove like a bat out of hell – and I am the greatest driver in the world, of course.

After briefings from the scientists and the head geologist, aptly named Professor Sparks, plus what administrators there were on Montserrat, we climbed back into the helicopter, put our lap straps back on and arranged our cameras. My eldest son, David, the great doer and organiser of our family who is a professional photographer, had chosen a super camera and given me a crash course on how to use it before I left. We were to be taken around Montserrat to see the damage for ourselves. To give us a better view, they took the sides off the beast and there we sat exposed to the clouds. Bowen and Bernie cunningly chose centre seats, so Ann, Dennis, our clerk and I were on the outside clinging to the helicopter roof with one hand and taking pictures with the other. I have to say that after an hour, my hand was locked into position and had to be prised off the helicopter roof, but those pictures were magnificent – they had to be. Looking down on the north of the island as we rose above St John's, we saw the tropical idyll of Montserrat. Neat houses of varying sizes in little villages with gardens overflowing with vegetation and flowers, but as we moved south, the landscape dramatically changed. At first, it looked like some farmers had been burning stubble and then, like a woodland fire, all the trees blackened and died. Then we noticed that the ground was covered with ash, and as we moved closer and closer to the Soufrière Hills, a lunar landscape was revealed. All grey and silver, no vegetation, just wipe-out. Bramble Airport, which used to bring the rich and famous to frolic in Montserrat, could barely be recognised with the runway deep under volcanic ash. We flew over Plymouth, the old capital, and saw derelict and burned-out houses standing forlorn in the ash and the old colonial governor's residence reduced to a shell. Weird to see such devastation made by nature alone.

One of the many scandals which emerged about Montserrat during our investigation was that all this had been predicted by a brilliant report, published in 1987 by two scientists Geoffrey Wadge and Michael Isaacs, entitled 'Volcanic Hazards from Soufrière Hills Volcano Montserrat'. Professor Sparks had told us that the report had anticipated many of the things which had happened. We learnt that the FCO had not seen the report, and Montserratian government ministers who had seen and presumably read the report in 1987 claimed that it had been 'blown away' in the hurricane of 1989, and everyone forgot it. Redevelopment of the island had taken place with £16.8 million of UK taxpayers' money, following the hurricane in all of those areas which Wadge and Isaacs had said were in most danger from the volcano. To add insult to injury, two months before the volcano became active again in

1994, a disaster preparedness manual had been published, making no mention of any volcano! Back home, my youngest son, who had done so much to help me get elected, was just setting out on a career as a geologist. I have learned so much from him about geology and the natural world and, with his brother, they have become a real resource for me.

We carried on uncovering a catalogue of inefficiency, complacency and self-interest, which had meant a total failure to protect the people of Montserrat who, if fit enough, had voted with their feet and got out, only to find that Antigua could not cope with them and the UK was very unwelcoming. There was a total lack of co-ordination and muddle on all fronts due to lousy administration over decades within Montserrat and from the UK government. It is to Clare Short's credit that she banged heads together and made progress in the delivery of aid and recognised very quickly the people who were trying to line their own pockets as a result of the disaster. Clare could make herself very unpopular at times, but I have always admired her for her forthrightness and fearlessness in telling things how they are. She hasn't climbed much further up the greasy pole of politics, of course. Too honest by far.

Bernie Grant was, I thought at the time, obsessed by which firms were getting the contracts for reconstruction and delivery of services on the island. Loud, ironic laughter had burst out of his huge frame when we were told that the contracts, like many DFID contracts, were going to Brown and Root, a big American company that dealt with everything from supplying tea urns to relief workers to massive reconstruction after disasters and war all over the world. Years later, I discovered that the same company, a subsidiary of Halliburton of Dick Cheney fame, was delivering all the needs of the people of Iraq after the war. This massive organisation makes trillions out of disaster and conflict. Bernie Grant knew. We just thought he had a bit of a bee in his bonnet.

The next morning, a personal disaster struck. We had a slightly later start, and I decided to have a leisurely shower and then sit out on the little yard outside my hotel room and read for half an hour before we mustered for more meetings with ministers in Antigua. A nice idea, in theory, if it wasn't for the gloom and the monkeys who feel obliged to come and keep you company and steal anything they can lay their hands on. Just as I stepped out of the shower, I heard the volcano blow, and I was determined to get a picture of the amazing mushroom of ash and sparks, which could be easily seen across the narrow strait between Antigua and Montserrat. Forgetting the shiny tiled floor, I dashed into the bedroom, stark naked and dripping wet, to grab my camera. I slid a few feet before landing flat on my face on the white tiles, banging my nose hard. As I reached for a towel to catch the blood which was now pouring from my nose onto the pristine white floor, a bird, a beautiful frigate bird, disorientated by the explosion, crashed into the plate glass window of my room, breaking its neck and causing blood to pour down the window. I sat on the floor, nursing my nose and laughing at the carnage. It looked as though ritual slaughter had been going on. The only good news is that I had not reached my beautiful camera so that at least was not injured. I summoned the poor maid to help clear up, and ice was found for my nose, which, as well as bleeding from within, had a large cut across the bridge, which I duly sealed up with butterfly sutures. I had bought an emergency medical kit with me in case it was needed, primarily for the others if they needed it, but I was the only person who used it, of course. I gave my room maid an extra big tip and spent the rest of the trip looking like I had been in a boxing bout the night before.

That evening, to cheer us up after a day of listening to government officials on Antigua professing ignorance of all sorts of things they should have known, Ann Clwyd, Dennis Canavan and I decided to have a meal in the restaurant on the local beach. It was straw-roofed and set on a platform over the shallows. Ann and I slipped into skirts for once, and the three of us watched the sunset over the Caribbean while we ate delicious local seafood. I always eat local food if I can on international development trips. I think eating what the people are used to cooking is the safest bet. I have never ever had a problem with food, and so far, Delhi Belly, Montezuma's Revenge and Gippy Tummy have never hit me. I did once get ill after flying home by Sabena Airlines, who no longer exist – enough said! The morning after our Caribbean night experience, both Ann and I had legs with measles! Our legs, already swollen from sitting in meetings in the heat, were now smothered in red spots from the sandflies coming up between the planks of the restaurant floor. We had forgotten all about insect repellent on the legs, exposed for the first time on that trip. It was trousers from then on. Imagine the sight of me with a plastered bruised nose and legs looking like spotted dick sponge pudding. One of the things I dislike about the tropics is the creaming that has to go on with sunscreen and insect repellent until you smell like a chemical factory and feel like flypaper. How ill-equipped we are to cope with these challenges coming from temperate climes.

That day we visited the poor souls who had been left by their families or chose to stay in Montserrat during the crisis. Many were elderly, and there was a high proportion of mentally and physically sick and disabled people. We were told that about 2000 people had stayed and we visited a group living in a church hall. There were a communal kitchen and tables and chairs for sitting to eat, but the 'living' accommodation for each family group was large pallets covered with mattresses, separated by an assortment of old curtains. One poor woman sat there staring into the curtain stroking a disabled and severely mentally handicapped large child who was lying on the bed chuntering and thrashing. The rest of the family had gone to Antigua, but she had felt she must stay with her daughter, who needed constant care. She was hopeful that the government would provide them with somewhere to live so that the family could be reunited.

Despite the crisis of the volcano, now into its third year, no new housing had been built for a number of reasons. Unaccountably the government of Montserrat had not asked for aid for new housing in the safe northern part of the island. They wanted government offices of course, like all good bureaucrats and, amazingly, a police station to police 2000 mainly elderly or sick people! Clare Short had refused, and in response to the request for a new police station, had made the famous remark, 'They will be asking for golden elephants next.' The opposition and many in my party were delighted that they had a 'gaffe' to exploit, but how right she was. Efforts were being made to compulsorily purchase the land in the north, which landowners were hanging on to, hoping to make a fortune. It was not a scenario filled with the milk of human kindness by any means. Meanwhile, the old women wiped the sweat away, and the few children left ran out into the churchyard to relieve themselves. More people, and there would surely have been a cholera outbreak.

The last day in Antigua was occupied by a public meeting in the centre of town in a low-roofed building with mostly open sides. The whole of Antigua had turned up, it seemed, to plea not just for the Montserratians but for everything under the sun for Antigua, which seemed pretty well close to paradise to me at the time compared with the fiery hell of Montserrat. That afternoon we were treated to a trip out to Nelson's Dockyard. It is difficult to believe but when we were at war with the French in the 18th century, the French had ships and a garrison on Guadeloupe, and the Brits had similar on Antigua. In a beautiful hidden harbour, we saw the entire garrison with all the naval workshops necessary to repair the sailing ships of the time. There were billets for the men on shore and shops and a pub, of course. The pièce de résistance was 'Lady Hamilton's House', which Nelson had built especially for her. He must have been so special, that man, for Lady Hamilton to undertake a precarious sea voyage across the Atlantic lasting weeks to see her lovely Horatio.

We left the Caribbean, not only determined to pursue the needs of the neglected people of Montserrat and to push for a sustainable development plan but to look at the muddle around the dependent territories generally, whose peoples were not regarded as citizens of the UK and yet were the direct responsibility of our Foreign

Office, with any aid necessary coming from the Department for International Development (DFID). Surely, we thought, we should regard these dependent territories as part of the UK but overseas, much in the same way as the French, where places like Guadeloupe are treated as 'departments' of France, and their people as full French citizens. In the course of that Labour Government, thanks to the hard work of that star politician Robin Cook, a truly British compromise was reached, and Montserrat and other dependencies are now called 'Overseas Territories'.

Chapter 10: Constituency Tales

1998 started with a visit to Kingston Parish Church for the Epiphany Service. This was a pleasure as well as a duty. I was brought up in a regular, church-going, Anglican family but had long since become agnostic. I nevertheless loved church liturgy and music. All Saints Church, Kingston, is an ancient church of Saxon foundation, with a coronation stone of its own in the churchyard where seven Anglo-Saxon kings were crowned long ago. It has a Scandinavian Frobenius Organ, which makes a stupendous sound and a choirmaster who is head of music at the local Tiffin's School. An evening at Kingston Parish Church is not to be missed.

Two days later, I was at Stringfellows Club with Diana Lamplugh, fundraising for the Susie Lamplugh Trust. Diana and Paul Lamplugh had lost their daughter Susie, an estate agent murdered by a client she was showing around a house. Her body has never been found, even though the police are fairly sure they have the man who did it, who is now in prison for other crimes. Diana and Paul were constituents of mine and founders of a trust to campaign for the safety of young people everywhere. They had persuaded Sir George Young, who had won the Private Members' Bill ballot in the previous session of parliament, to take a Bill to register minicabs in London. Unbelievably, at that time, anyone could buy an old car and without any checks pose as a minicab service on the streets of London. Many crimes had been committed on young women and men, and in Kingston, we had a case of a rapist released from prison one day, buying an old car, and going out the following night to offer lifts outside a club. He raped a girl passenger that night. The Bill had got nowhere in 1997, despite much hard work by Sir George Young backed by Simon Hughes and others. Diana and Paul Lamplugh decided to try again, and I was roped in to help.

We also persuaded the 'It' girl Tamara Beckwith to come and be photographed getting in and out of cars to try and liven the campaign up a bit and draw it to the attention of younger people. Tamara was a great sport and a huge help. Irrepressible and quite naughty, at primary school in Kew, she and my daughter had been inseparable collaborators in mischief-making, and although they had been apart for secondary school, they had kept vaguely in touch. The Bill's main opposition came from MPs supporting the black cab lobby in London, who did not want competition from less well-trained drivers who had not done 'The Knowledge', the famous course which enables black cabbies to take you wherever you want to go without hesitation. The Bill eventually passed after many parliamentary dodges and procedures by the enemy to defeat it, engineered mainly by the LibDem whips led by a skilled and masterful Paul Tyler. Interesting to ponder on what will happen to 'The Knowledge' now that sat navs and mobile apps have arrived.

Transport continued to dominate the winter with the continuation of the Terminal 5 inquiry for Heathrow. Aircraft noise and pollution from traffic to and from Heathrow is the dominant issue in Richmond Park constituency. Summer garden peace is destroyed, lessons are disrupted in schools and sleep is disturbed all over the area as the night flight quota rumbles overhead. In fact, every transport minister in the Commons and Lords has been invited to come and stay with me (and my family) to have the Heathrow experience. They have all declined, and T5 is up and running, with the threat of more expansion at that infamous airport to follow in the form of a third runway. I spoke to the T5 inquiry on three occasions because it went on for four long years. The length of these inquiries is ludicrous, but the idea that we can control global warming and all its consequences without curtailing air transport is also ludicrous. My successor and all of the campaign groups continue the battle.

During the campaign for the 1992 General Election, I came across a small business operation in a basement on Richmond Green. Perhaps I was delivering leaflets? I cannot remember. It turned out to be my first encounter with someone who was a pretty aggressive and scary character at that time. No lover of wealthy Richmond Green, it was John Bird – not the actor – who quickly told me about his project to produce a street newspaper to be sold by unemployed and homeless people as a social enterprise. That newspaper was The Big Issue, and John Bird was its founder. He is now an esteemed colleague of mine in the House of Lords, with many successful social enterprises and businesses, all encouraging the less fortunate in our society to get back on their feet. Orphaned as a five-year-old, he was brought up in children's homes and did several terms in prison for petty theft before turning himself around and using the education he had received in prison to start a small business. I came across him several times when I was in the Commons after he moved to larger premises outside Richmond, but I was always rather pleased to think he started in my constituency.

Another interesting constituent was associated with the name of the constituency – Richmond Park. I had a meeting, early on in my first term as a member of parliament, with a businessman called Daniel Hearsum, who had bought from the Crown Estate the lease of a beautiful but very dilapidated house in Richmond Park called Pembroke Lodge, once the home of the liberal Russell family. Its previous owners had run a café there, and Daniel wanted to make it into an upmarket entertaining and conference centre. To do this, he had for several years lived in the upper part of the house with his family, but was trying to persuade the Crown Estate to allow him to renovate the large cottage in the grounds as a family house to enable him to use the upper part of the house as another entertaining room, and also to house his collection of memorabilia of the Russell family, of whom he was a great fan. I, and the LibDem-controlled council in Richmond at the time, supported him and still do. Pembroke Lodge is now one of the finest conference and entertainment centres in the south of England, which has to be booked years ahead for weddings and parties. Daniel and the Liberal Democrats have remained firm friends ever since, and the facility is frequently used for their party events. Daniel is also creating a Heritage Centre in the park nearby, where people can learn about the natural history of the park. He has even further ambitions to expand to show the history of the park: before it was enclosed for Royal hunting, there were tiny villages and workers' cottages, the outline of which can be seen on some aerial views.

One of my grandsons is the proud owner of a George the First penny, which he found in the park some years ago and was identified by the experts behind the scenes at The Antiques Roadshow when it came to the park in 2013. Probably a week's wages for some poor farm labourer, they said, lost until found 300 years later. I hope his family did not go hungry that week.

Light relief in February 1998 was provided by HM the Queen, who had decided to hold a couple of evening receptions at Buckingham Palace so that she and her family could meet members of the House of Commons. Keith and I trooped along in best suits, meeting Labour MP Ben Bradshaw in the courtyard, furious because male partners of male MPs had not been invited, the palace still resisting the new political correctness (and fairness). He came, though. We were all given drinks in one of those incredible rooms at Buck House that feel like a film set. Then we were announced one by one as we went into supper, greeted by the Queen and Prince Philip, the latter commenting that I must have an easy job as MP for Richmond Park because only his cousin, Princess Alexandra, and her family lived there. I reminded him there were lots of deer too. My team subsequently wondered if we could get LibDem stickers for the rumps of the deer, but sadly decided against it. The Queen and other members of the family circled around as we ate our supper, and we were warned that if the Queen came up to our group, she would decide the topic of conversation, and we were not to change the subject. We stood in fear and trepidation with Adrian Saunders, one of the southwest LibDem MPs, and his wife as the Queen approached. No medical viva had been as tense as this. What would she say?

'Hello, where do you represent?' she said to Adrian Saunders.

'Oh, err, Torbay, Ma'am, in Devon.'

'Really. I went there once in the Royal Yacht. We were promised a wonderful view in the morning, but when we got up, it was just *thick fog.*'

Adrian, blushing red and feeling totally responsible for the royal disappointment, half bowed and said, 'I'm terribly sorry, Ma'am.'

We half expected, hoped even, that he would be sent to the Tower, but she moved away with a smile to 'get to know' someone else. Poor Adrian was often reminded of his conversation with the monarch. A lovely idea, but why oh why does our Head of State have to be kept, generation after generation, in a gilded cage with no real contact with the people. Let's hope it will be easier for William if he ever makes it to the throne.

Soon after this, the Select Committee for International Development was Africa bound on our very first fact-finding trip during the investigation into Conflict Prevention and Conflict Resolution.

Chapter 11: Into Africa

This Select Committee trip was a much bigger and longer affair than the dash to Montserrat six months before. The main purpose of these trips is to see where tax payers' money is going and whether it is wisely spent. We took evidence from all sorts of people and organisations before we went and had decided to do a study of a country which had emerged from terrible conflict such as Uganda, recovering from the Idi Amin years; Kenya, which was one of the stars of the African continent but thought due to poor governance to be sliding towards catastrophe; and Rwanda which was still reeling from civil war and the terrible genocide of Tutsi people by the Hutu, when the world and UN peacekeepers had stood by and watched.

The whole select committee was going on this trip, and we were such an interesting group: Bowen Wells, our gentle, humorous and hugely experienced Chairman; Labour MPs Bernie Grant, Dennis Canavan and Ann Clwyd (who had been with me in Montserrat); and Piara Kabra, the MP for Southall where I had worked for years before becoming an MP. Piara was the first Sikh to be elected to parliament; he was frail, elderly and very deaf, so that he frequently had to be looked after because he never heard the instructions but knew an awful lot about an awful lot. There were two Tories. Andrew Robathan, ex-army and keen on efficient organisation who was constantly frustrated by the relaxed attitudes to time and management in Africa. I nicknamed him 'Action Man'. He was a great asset and amazingly knew the name of every bird in Africa. The other Andrew was Andrew Rowe, a tall, elegant, old-fashioned Conservative with a firm and devout Christian faith who worked for and encouraged many third world charities. Two young women made up the group. One was Tess Kingham, who had had twins just after being elected to parliament in the great New Labour landslide; she had an NGO background and was a huge asset. She became a close friend during her four years in parliament but stood down after one term, totally disillusioned with New Labour and wanting to be with her family – a great loss. The other was Oona King, Labour member for Bethnal Green and Bow. Lively, argumentative, all-singing, dancing (and swearing) Oona. She would often descend into the hotel lobby, always the last to appear, and astonish everyone with a pristine white, jewelled salwar kameez, to spend the day in a dirty Land Rover, grubbing around village projects. She sure wowed the locals, who thought she was royalty.

There is something to be said for Oona's approach. Our visit was probably the most exciting thing that happened to the people in the villages we visited, and she provided that star quality. It complimented them too. I loved Oona, still do. After our first trip, she insisted on calling me 'Mum' because I was always worrying about her, providing aspirins or Dioralyte or lending money when she had run out of cash to buy artefacts! Our committee clerks were Yusuf Asad, son of my constituents in Kingston, and Janet Hughes. These clerks are the stars of any trip with parliamentarians. They are responsible for everything and get blamed for everything. They take all the notes and write up the reports. Yusuf and Janet were brilliant, patient, efficient, humorous, discreet – I have run out of complimentary adjectives.

Our first stop was Uganda, and we arrived at Entebbe after an overnight flight, business class from Heathrow. Is there anything more enjoyable? I often wonder. Plenty of legroom and feet up space for sleep after a decent dinner with wine. Luxurious limbo, with no phones, no family, no constituents' problems to fret about. Our only task was to swot up on the briefings we had been given by the clerks before we left. We had a mere 350 pages of notes on debt, trade, the position of women, conflict and geography and demography of the three countries we were to visit. Needless to say, sleep soon took care of that, and we had to dip frantically in and out of the notes as we travelled around. What a mountain of paper we brought home. Each UK government department in the three countries had also prepared briefs for us, as had each department of the three countries we visited and each individual project leader. I resolved always to take an extra empty bag on any journey in future. Some of it got read; I cannot say all. The clerks would have read every word.

On the drive from Entebbe Airport to Kampala, I pondered why every village we passed through had one or two huts outside, piled high with oblong wooden boxes of all sizes from tiny to huge. 'AIDS epidemic', said the Ugandan civil servant accompanying us. 'They are coffin makers. It's the best business to be in nowadays.' In 1998 the AIDS crisis was only just unfolding. In the UK, it was mainly confined to certain groups, but here in Africa, it was rampant and causing all sorts of problems for communities that we were to discover.

Our first day in Uganda involved a long 3½ hour journey to Mbale in the east of Uganda because we took a wrong turning off the great Mombasa-Kampala-Kigali highway, which is Africa's artery, running from the coast to the heart of Africa. It is also notorious for its sex workers, who live along the highway to serve the truckers taking loads into the hinterland. It has been dubbed the 'AIDS Highway' by the NGOs.

The detour gave us a wonderful view of Uganda. Neat villages with traditional round huts with large straw hats for roofs gave the countryside an idyllic air and looked just like those pictures in school geography books entitled 'A Ugandan Village'. Children poured out as we passed through and waved and laughed. The roads are lined with people walking in Uganda, usually with heavy water containers or laden baskets. Walking to the wells and back, walking to the fields and back, walking to school and back. Everyone walks everywhere! The wheel does not feature because there are no roads, except the one we were on. The vegetation grows so furiously, sometimes three crops each year, so that even a basic track gets overgrown in a couple of weeks. So rural Ugandans carry on walking until their lives' end. The towns we passed through were not so beautiful. We were to learn of the migration of people to the towns and cities for work, just as happened in the 19th century in the UK. These people have to live in stinking slums with open sewer trenches running past their shacks, made from any bit of corrugated iron or board they can find. Nevertheless, the children still ran out to wave, laughing and shouting. You learn a lot about the human spirit in Africa.

We had a planned stop in a village on our way and tumbled out in our slacks and shirts, except for Oona, resplendent as ever and looking like a princess in her snow-white salwar kameez. It was a good job that she, at least, had made an effort. We were greeted by massed singing and dancing by hundreds of people making a *huge* noise which lasted whilst we were given Coca-Cola or Fanta to drink and introduced to all the head people in the area. I was to learn that Coca-Cola gets to those parts of the world that nothing else can reach. Wherever I go in the third world, they may be short of medical supplies and condoms in particular (the story of one condom per man per year in Africa was absolutely true and has not improved much). But you can always buy Coca-Cola if you have any money. Why, oh why, can't they market condoms and Coca-Cola together? I have suggested this on many occasions back in the UK, but there is no interest. My cynical mind says that condoms might put people off buying Coca-Cola, and even more cynically, condoms might prevent a disease, which is now a huge earner for the pharmaceutical industry in the form of anti-retroviral drugs used to treat AIDS.

That great leader of the Western World, George W. Bush, had pumped billions of dollars into the global fund to treat AIDS and related diseases which were being spent on drugs. At the same time that devout Christian also stopped funds going to UNFPA (United Nations Population Fund), which had to stop their programmes of sexual health, education and condom distribution because they also advised about safe abortion in countries where unsafe abortion is one of the main causes of maternal death. What a fine man is Dubya? All this is in the future, however.

After we had enjoyed the show in the village, we were entertained by a group of women who had drawn cartoons to illustrate their day's work and more cartoons illustrating the men's day. The women rise at dawn and start the long walk for water. Then they trudge back to the village, where they wake the little ones, give them some food. They then prepare the husband's food before waking him up. He eats breakfast and then goes to sit under a tree with the other men where they discuss 'important business' – this said with great irony. The women then clean the compound and sweep the floors, the dust forming beautiful and artistic swirls as they do so. They then go to the fields for several hours until it is time for the older children to come back from school and the evening meal has to be prepared. During this time, the men take a well-earned rest during the afternoon – talking to your friends, the women said, is very exhausting! There was loud laughter at this point and nods of agreement from the men who were enjoying this presentation as much as we were. The tale went on of woman's toil and man's idleness. It was good to see feminism alive and well in Uganda.

A formal presentation then took place. We handed over the obligatory gift from the House of Commons, and the mayor of the village moved forward bearing a huge live turkey! This was their present to their honoured guests from England. We all shrank back and pushed forward DFID's man in Uganda to receive our gift. He was a tall, beetling man with specs on the end of his nose and looked a bit of a turkey himself standing there nearly obscured by feathers. It was not one of the most elegant moments in his career, but it must be one of the most memorable. Bowen Wells, with enormous tact and grace, suggested that we should donate the turkey for a special feast for the local people that night after we had left. This was accepted. Poor turkey!

We saw many brilliant projects in Uganda, which, under the government of President Museveni, was making great strides despite enormous problems. The Tories, especially Bowen Wells, insisted that the government was rotten because it was a single-party state, but you had to understand its problem. Museveni had decided that allowing political parties after the Amin years would mean the country dividing along tribal lines, which is seen still in so many African countries. He had decreed that there would be four-yearly elections to the local village and town councils, who would elect their representatives from that body to the regional government, who again would elect from that body to the national government. I suppose there was corruption within the system, but it seemed to be working so far as a bottom-up, representative system could, and they had a much higher proportion of women in national government than we did in the UK, despite Tony Blair and his all-women shortlists. We certainly heard no complaints about the system whilst we were in Uganda but got lobbied by exiled Ugandans when we got back to the UK. It caused a lot of discussion over dinner about our democracy and whether we should always try to get other countries in different stages of development to adopt it. On the whole, the Tories thought we should – they quoted Churchill, saying that democracy is not perfect, but it's the best system we have got. Maybe for us at our stage of development with a high proportion of educated citizens, that applies, but not for every developing country. Surely, they must be allowed to work out their own salvation as we had done?

We saw very impressive health projects in Uganda. Museveni and his government had recognised the threat of AIDS very early on and put into action a countrywide prevention scheme. All schools received sex education and were taught about AIDS and the dangers of unprotected sex. We saw the boys of one grammar school in Kampala enact a play about a local Romeo who loved all girls as they loved him. He refused to listen to his friends' warnings, and so eventually, he died a terrible death from AIDS, trying to warn them of his foolishness. It would have translated well into some of our schools, we thought! AIDS patients themselves in the early stages of the disease went round the village health centres teaching about prevention. There were no drugs available then, as there are now, except to prevent the transmission of AIDS to babies when mothers gave birth.

There had been huge problems coming to terms with the problems of female circumcision or female genital mutilation (FGM). It happened all over Africa and was certainly acknowledged by the doctors there. Nobody wanted to talk about it, though, and governments have banned it, but still, it goes on. I was to come back to this issue over and over again much later on in the Commons and the Lords

Uganda was trying hard to improve the health of its people, but clean water and sewage disposal, which are the key to health – more important than doctors and drugs – were still hard to come by. Nevertheless, progress was being made, not just by aid projects from foreign countries but by the Ugandans themselves. Education was a better story. Uganda was committed to universal primary education, and the evidence was everywhere. Parents still had to pay for the rather quaint English style school clothes which we saw children wearing all over the country. The tiniest hut would produce several little ones, all bandbox clean in their uniforms, going off to school.

We went to a teachers' centre out in the bush where I came to grief. After listening to the work that was being done there, I had asked for the loo before setting back on a bumpy journey to the next centre. The teachers had gone, and I thought everyone knew I had also nipped to the lavatory. When I emerged, all I could see were our two Land Rovers hurtling across the landscape, already about a mile away. There I was, stuck outside a deserted school building with no one around. Half of our party had gone that day to visit Gulu in the north, where the dreaded Lord's Resistance Army abducted people and children to fight their disgusting war on the borders of Sudan. I tried to put this out of my head. I had no mobile phone (Bernie was the only person in those days who had such a thing), and it was late afternoon. I felt a bit worried but decide to walk down the hill towards a tiny group of huts at the bottom of the hill, where I hoped to get help.

A man came up to meet me from the village and immediately

realised what had happened. He was one of the teachers at the centre we had visited. He had the brilliant idea of getting me onto a 'moto-moto' to take me to where he knew our party had gone. I had to trust him. The skinniest boy I have ever seen was called up. He had a very old push-bike with a saddlebag frame which had a padded and fringed cushion fixed to it. This was it, a Ugandan rural taxi. It was better than the wooden bikes children ride all over Africa. This poor child pedalled me about four miles to the next stop. I had to get off on the hills and walk – I must have been five times his weight. As we neared the school, I saw the Land Rovers and a frantic Janet, the clerk who had realised too late that I was missing. Children poured out to meet my bicyclist saviour, and dozens of them ran alongside cheering as I arrived triumphantly in the schoolyard, still perched on my fringed cushion. There was then an argument about how much to pay my moto boy. I was all for giving him every Ugandan shilling I had, so grateful was I for my deliverance, but the elders insisted he was paid the going rate – a pittance, in other words. I was not allowed to intervene but was later given a telling off by the clerks for not staying where I was until they realised I was left behind and returned for me. All very well thought I. You were not the lonely soul on the Ugandan hillside with night falling. Ah well, another lesson learned. I have never forgotten that ride and the strength of that boy child who pedalled me to safety.

The Ugandan economy was in a very parlous state in 1998. We visited a sugar estate: much tea is grown there, but one of the biggest problems is dire poverty, especially amongst women who, for many reasons, are the sole supporter of their families. In Kampala, we visited a poverty reduction project based on microcredit, of which I was to become a great fan, as I learned about the issues in development. Microcredit was thought up by a Bangladeshi, Muhammad Yunus, whose birthday party I was to attend whilst at a conference in New York a couple of years later. He started lending small amounts of money primarily to women in Bangladesh to enable them to start small businesses to support their families. He found not only that it was hugely popular and successful, but his borrowers did not default – there was a 98 per cent repayment rate. Here in Uganda, DFID had started a similar scheme, and it was a roaring success. It was here that I got the proverbial answer to a proverbial question. I asked one woman what she would do if she could have anything in the world. A trip to America? Clothes, a car, a television?

'A cow', she said. With a cow, she could feed her children, and with the funds from selling surplus milk, she would send them to school. They have values, these people. The day before, I had marvelled at a man living in a slum on the borders of Kampala, where we had stopped briefly. He had educated all of his children because of his fine 'business'. His business had started when he had built himself a bike out of bits of scrap he had found around Kampala over the years. Every morning he rode the 30 miles to Entebbe Airport – a long, long way on a homemade bike. At the airport, he collected all the newspapers from the planes that had arrived overnight and cycled back to his hut where his wife had the flat iron heated up on the fire. Together they ironed and refolded the newspapers, and then off he went into Kampala and stood in the market until he had sold them all. He was extremely proud of his business, and he was a true entrepreneur – Alan Sugar be proud. My children got rather sick of this story when I got back. I used it to demonstrate to them that with energy and enterprise, they would never lack food or education. Living near Heathrow has to be a bonus, let's face it.

On the macro level, Uganda shared its problems with the other countries we were to visit. The need for debt relief was one, and the other was a lack of megawatts. Without electricity, no one will invest. We sat through some long and pretty boring meetings about trade and manufacturing and energy supplies, all very necessary to know about. We visited the Jinja dam to see the Owen Falls hydro-electric power project, which was nearly at the end of a refurbishment financed jointly by the World Bank, the Commonwealth Development Corporation and DFID. It had been a huge job with escalating costs, and there remained doubts that it would be maintained properly if it was kept in public ownership.

We saw a great deal of evidence in Africa to suggest that public ownership, whilst being ideologically a 'good thing', in fact, led to decaying infrastructure and a gross waste of international funds. After a few visits, I became a convert to privatisation for these projects, much to the delight of Bowen Wells and his fellow Tories. That trip was made even more special by lunch at the Jinja Yacht Club on Lake Victoria and a walk to see the source of the White Nile out of the lake head. That night, having pre-dinner drinks on the High Commissioner's lawn, I realised just how much I was enjoying myself.

So Uganda was our example of an up-and-coming African country, making great strides towards democracy and prosperity, developing largely at peace and healing wounds after the tribal wars in the desperate days of Idi Amin's time. Who are we to think that we must insist on our version of democracy? Uganda's version of democracy was strange, but surely it should evolve to match local needs. I was to reflect on this a great deal during my time in parliament. In 2009 I had to return to Uganda to present one of my All-Party Parliamentary Group's papers to an international conference of parliamentarians there. Kampala had certainly improved, but progress had slowed as Museveni clung to power in his one-party state, which sadly is the pattern all over Africa.

The committee then moved on to Kenya; a stable, prosperous country thought to be going downhill due to corrupt administration. The Nairobi Safari Club hotel was prosperous enough. Full of ex-pats and business people living the high life, although outside its doors children were begging and trying to sell single cigarettes to the occupants of cars stopped at traffic lights. We were told the crime rate was high too; although swept around as we were in High Commission Land Rovers, it did not affect us, of course! That first day in Kenya, we toured around government departments listening to various ministers and civil servants put a gloss on everything for the visitors from the UK. One story that sticks in my mind is that of the Mombasa Highway, which is the road running from the coast right through Kenya and on to the centre of Africa, the 'AIDS Highway' of Uganda. The World Bank had financed a new road, but sadly with the first heavy flooding, it had been washed away. There was an argument about who should repair this essential bit of infrastructure because it turned out that the World Bank money had been pocketed by officials, and a contractor had just laid a thin layer of tarmac on the highway to make it look good, with no proper foundation. So, it washed away. The worst floods in a generation after a long drought meant that Kenya was facing many very genuine problems of poverty, even though it was not regarded as a heavily indebted country. Forty-eight per cent of the population were still below the poverty line, and we could see that malnutrition, malaria and AIDS were rife.

There followed a weekend break from visiting officials and projects – actually much needed during a two-week trek. We were flown in a small aircraft up to the Samburu region, where we were to overnight in the Samburu Serena Lodge Hotel. On the flight up, we saw the Rift Valley and the Aberdare Mountains, and even Mount Kenya topped with snow. A lake edged in pink turned out to be flamingos feeding at the edge of the water—such a stunningly beautiful landscape. There is nothing like a small light aircraft for getting a good view of the countryside.

On arrival, we were immediately driven off to visit a major project run by our own Department for International Development in a primary school and teacher advisory centre. This was followed by a game drive in the Samburu National Park where, yes, I saw my very first herd of elephants come down to the river to give the little ones a bedtime bath and feed. A truly wonderful sight.

After dinner in the hotel, we went to a lecture on conservation links. This guy said that too many were surviving, and it was not sustainable – he was referring to human beings too. Education was not practicable here, so the tribal people were used for decoration around the hotel in Samburu dress, for tourists to photograph.

Some of them, the privileged ones presumably, became servants in the hotel. I felt outraged – this was worse than Schweitzer and his 'younger brother' theory. Here was a westerner advocating that education was a waste of time for the Samburu and that they should be kept as far as possible like a species in a zoo for people to wonder at. Had I misunderstood? He did not mention the position of women or the advisability of promoting family planning. They were just secondary chapters, not to be considered. The debate raged amongst us into the night.

The next morning breakfast was served on the beach of a wide muddy river, not the 'great grey-green greasy Limpopo River, best beloved, where the elephant got his trunk', but something similar, and it was certainly where the crocodiles came for tea and breakfast. The Samburu men, in full regalia, stood on the beach near the water's edge to hit the crocs on the nose as they smelt the cooking and came along for food. We were served bacon and eggs, with all the English trimmings, from silver dishes, sitting at tables covered with good English damask cloths. Champagne was served, too - the true safari experience!

That morning was free, and I declined another safari trek (sad, they saw a lion) and sat on the veranda outside my room, writing up notes and reading the pages and pages of information provided by the organisers. I was bombed by a hornbill and plagued incessantly by monkeys who will steal everything they can lay their hands on, just for the hell of it – I don't suppose they had much use for a Bic biro anyway. At lunchtime, one of them came to the table and stole my bread roll. I swear it was the same one perched up in the rafters who peed on me as we walked out to get the next plane to fly us to Kisumu on Lake Victoria.

We were greeted in Kisumu by a BBC2 team who were filming the trip and had come out ahead of us. They informed us with great excitement that Kisumu was a hell hole and the mozzies were as big as cockroaches. And so it was. Lake Victoria at Kisumu is almost completely silted up with Water Hyacinth, a non-native plant that had arrived in Kenya via a missionary in the 19th century. He brought it from South America, so the story goes because his wife thought it was beautiful and wanted it in her garden pond in Kenya. Sounds a bit rich. The wretched plant had done so well with its thick fibrous roots and, without a natural enemy in Africa, had single-handedly closed the port of Kisumu because no boat could get through the dense mass of roots. The still, stagnant water was the perfect environment for Africa's greatest enemy, the malaria mosquito. When I got back to the UK, I asked the Royal Botanic Gardens, Kew, in my constituency, about it. The problem had been picked up, and botanists were working on the case somewhere. I later heard that a beetle had been introduced to eat the stuff, and the results were promising. When we were there, however, all they could do was use some of it as hemp for baskets, chairs and tables, but with few customers for furniture and artefacts, little of the stuff was being used.

The only hotel, The Sunset, was also the local brothel, be it somewhat high class, and the bar was full of exotic sex workers, thick makeup, stilettos, the lot. The mosquitoes on the walls everywhere were indeed huge, and I wondered if I could defend myself against so many. Despite the giant mosquitoes, my long avoidance routine held good, and I was unscathed. Our rooms were away from the main building, and after dinner, we all opted for an early night before the next day's round of visits. Clutching my key – I was assured that my luggage was already in my room – I marched across the garden and up two flights of concrete stairs. The key would not work. I shook and hammered but to no avail. I had to go back to reception and fight my way through the girls to the desk and seek help. I had gone to the wrong block.

The next morning, a male member of our group was relating how one of the girls must have fancied him and had spent ages trying to get at his 'gorgeous' body by rattling the key and trying to get in. Was he disappointed when I told him it was me?

He was relieved the next morning that he had escaped the

attention of the Kisumu girls when we visited an AIDS project in the town and saw the relentless spread of the disease through the population. The whole day was spent visiting projects, a pedal pump being the most notable way to get clean water using alternative technology. We also made our first visit to a Marie Stopes International clinic, doing amazing work with the women of Kisumu. Marie Stopes is a family planner's hero NGO, having fought for contraception to become acceptable in the UK in the 1920s. I am a great fan of the organisation that now bears her name. They do the most amazing work in clean, bright clinics, run with identical efficiency in all the countries I have visited. I could easily have walked in and started doctoring, having worked for them in the UK.

That evening we flew back to Nairobi, and, despite the fatigue, we were entertained royally by the High Commissioner in his beautiful residence in the diplomatic quarter. We wandered the gardens and argued about what we had seen so far and what we knew was to come – the depression and horrors of Rwanda, still in the throes of civil war and genocide. The conflict in Rwanda was very recent, just four years earlier and still wracked by killings when we visited.

Rwandan society consists of the Hutu, who are the majority, the Tutsi, and a tiny minority of Twa. The Tutsis, however, had always been the ruling class until after independence in 1959, when the Hutu, supported by France and Belgium, dominated a one-party state. At this time, many Tutsis had fled Rwanda and lived in exile in Uganda, where in the 1980s, they formed the Rwandan Patriotic Front, supported by President Museveni of Uganda. The RPF tried to invade Rwanda in 1990 but failed, and subsequently, a power-sharing settlement was arrived at between the Hutu and the RPF. This was shattered when the Hutu president's plane was shot down by persons unknown. The Hutu staged a coup and ordered the systematic slaughter of Tutsis in Rwanda, using radio broadcasts to whip up hatred and encourage relatives, neighbours and friends to turn upon the 'cockroaches' in society, meaning the Tutsi. Over a period of three months, nearly one million people were killed by machetes, knives and guns. They were shown no mercy. They were killed in schools and churches where they had dashed to try to find sanctuary. The RPF, led by Paul Kagame, who had been in hiding on the borders in an earth bunker which we visited on a subsequent visit to Rwanda, invaded his country and stopped the mass killings, although some killings were continuing somewhere every day in Rwanda. He set up a government in Kigali under a power-sharing agreement with Hutu and Tutsi holding office. Kagame, however, was the President and still is.

We were driven to the Hôtel des Mille Collines – the only hotel in Kigali. My first impression was of furtiveness and depression and, yes, palpable fear. The bell boys in the hotel sat in the darkest part of the corridors and never looked you in the eye. They had learned that over the terrible years they had been through. A poem I learnt as a child kept roaming around my head whilst I was there – Kipling's *Song of the Little Hunter*.

> *'Ere Mor the Peacock flutters, ere the Monkey People cry,*
>
> *Ere Chil the Kite swoops down a furlong sheer,*
>
> *Through the Jungle very softly flits a shadow and a sigh,*
>
> *He is Fear, O Little Hunter, he is Fear!'*

We were told that everyone was afraid and could no longer trust anyone. The Tutsi who had fled to the Congo had been pursued by Hutu Interahamwe and killed there. Many had returned as a consequence but were still expecting death at any moment.

We went to the government building, which was a windowless shell without water or electricity. Nevertheless, the assembly was there to meet us, and President Kagame addressed us. I think we were all bowled over by his grace and determination – a truly great man who had endured years of living rough before coming in to take control. He had established a police force and reopened schools and clinics. We were very welcome because the UK had supported them from the early days and was much respected; Clare Short, in particular, was singled out for praise. DFID was concentrating on education which is still benefiting the people of Rwanda. Sometimes we saw very worthwhile interventions, and this was one. They needed typewriters and photocopiers and a new generator until they could get power lines up again. It was a sobering experience to see people coping in such surroundings. Kagame had even insisted that women should be very prominent in his government and held many key posts. This was made easier in a way because so many of the men in Rwanda had been slaughtered, but women are still in an equal position to men in Rwanda.

We were taken to genocide 'sites', of course. One, in particular, had been a school on top of a hill where women and children had fled for safety only to be followed by the Hutu who slaughtered them as they lay down protecting their babies and children. The government had decided to leave the bodies as they were to remind people of the horrors. It was a hot, windy place, and I remember the strange musty smell there and countless little bodies under adult bodies. It was heart-wrenching. Later that day, we went to an orphanage for children of the genocide, and as I stood listening to the carers there tell us their plans for the children, I realised that a small hand had been put into mine and was clutching it tightly.

I looked down and smiled, but the little girl did not look at me or speak. One of the carers told me that they had managed to piece together her story. As a toddler, she had been shielded by her dead mother's body but had crawled out when the killers had gone and joined a string of survivors heading out of Rwanda towards Congo. She held on to the nearest hand as they trudged through the forest for days. She eventually found her father, but following another attack, she had lost him and just clutched the hand of the nearest adult and kept walking. She had never been heard to utter a sound even though she was now about six years old. When she was brought to the orphanage as people returned to Rwanda, she continued to hold the hand of any adult she was near, and I had been privileged to be in contact with this brave little girl. The orphanage had even managed to trace her father, but he had remarried, and his new wife did not want the murdered wife's child. I have never been able to get that child out of my head. She is a constant reminder of how fortunate my children and grandchildren are. There were thousands of children in orphanages and child-headed households in the Rwanda of 1998, four years after the genocide, many with similar stories. It was just one of the many challenges facing Paul Kagame.

A challenge that had not occurred to me before this visit was how an embryo government dealt with all the NGOs and UN organisations that flood into an area in their huge Land Rovers, laden with well-meaning projects and ideas. It takes a strong leader to accept help and not let it overwhelm. One quite ridiculous incident was experienced in a village project set up by the aid workers of the charity World Vision. They had encouraged and helped survivors of the genocide to write down their grievances and accusations against neighbours and erstwhile friends who had attacked them. A large wooden cross had been erected in the centre of the village, and the people were encouraged to nail their grievances to the Cross of Jesus, who would forgive the sins of their neighbours and make the village whole again. World Vision has an evangelical style.

Rather more effective, and due to the shortage of lawyers, Kagame had set up village 'courts' called Gacaca, where the men from that village who had committed these murders were brought and questioned, tried and sentenced by their neighbours. We watched this in action, and I must say it was impressive. The men convicted of the worst murders were sent to prisons like warehouses, with only enough bunks for half the inmates, so they changed over every twelve hours and stood outside. They all wore pink pyjamas! It was in one of these prisons, four years later on a follow-up visit, that Tom Clarke MP, who had declined to visit the gorillas a few days before because of his blood pressure, faced 2000 convicted génocidaires and gave a brave and impromptu address of encouragement to them all.

On that second visit, we saw a transformed Rwanda. Order had been restored, and the NGOs were less active. The government was functional, and Paul Kagame was determined to make Rwanda the high-tech centre of Africa – which it is becoming. In such a tiny country with a huge population, I was delighted that much emphasis had been put on maternal health and family planning – not easy in a predominantly Catholic country. It was working, however, and family size has continued to fall. It fell steadily from 8.21 children in 1968 to 3.81 children per woman in 2017. As a consequence, more women stay in full-time education and join the workforce. I returned to Rwanda in 2018 for an international conference on family planning and could not believe the further progress that country has made in 25 years since the genocide: education for all children up to secondary level and many carrying on after that, a beautifully organised health network from the health ministry down to the smallest village, delivering public health messages and family planning. I feel great hope that despite its huge population and tiny surface area, Rwanda will prosper as Botswana has done. Plans were laid to encourage investment, particularly in high-tech industries, and the places we visited were incredibly well-maintained and clean. Everywhere, the haunted faces we saw post-genocide had been replaced by smiling, relaxed people, all hoping for a better future. There are criticisms of President Kagame. Is he suppressing opposition, and will he follow in the footsteps of other liberators of their countries like Mugabe in Zimbabwe? I think not. He has huge numbers of women involved at every level of government and administration, which I think will make the difference. We shall see.

Soon after returning from Africa, I was invited with the other spokespeople for international development to 'meet' Nelson Mandela in South Africa House. Not a meeting exactly, but we listened to him speak and then had the thrill of actually shaking hands with that great man who had endured so much and yet had maintained his love of his fellow men and bore no grudges.

Chapter 12: Domes

The weather back home was quite a shock to get used to after a couple of weeks in Africa. The day Norman Baker, Liberal Democrat MP for Lewes, and I visited the Dome, or the site on The Thames on which they were building the Millennium Dome, there was thick mud, freezing temperatures and horizontal rain, the sort my family used to battle against during family holidays in Wales. Norman, who very early on was developing a reputation for tracking down government waste, was furious with the whole project. Romantic old me, having had my suggestion of 'Homes, not Domes' rejected as a party theme for the millennium – yes, there was a housing shortage then too – tried to imagine the finished project and was quite impressed.

The Dome itself would be a magnificent structure, and I remembered my joy as a child when we were taken to the Festival of Britain and naively expected the reaction to the Dome to be similar to the 'Dome of Discovery', the centrepiece of the Festival. I suppose in the fifties we were not used to television and computers and foreign travel for all, so we were in a state of wonderment over the festival on the South Bank, so soon after the deprivations of the war years. The Dome could never have succeeded in today's cynical and sophisticated society. Visiting the exhibition in 2000 to listen to schoolchildren from Richmond sing and dance in a competition, I found it very uninspiring inside. On that icy day two years before, my wonderful vision was replaced by one memory only, that of a talking wheelie-bin following me from the drinks area to the stage area where the children from my constituency were waiting to perform. I never found out what the wheelie bins were for because, like all MPs, I was due back in my constituency for something or another half an hour later.

1998 was an extraordinary year. The great Jubilee 2000 campaign to relieve the debt of the world's poorest countries got underway, and I travelled up to Birmingham with Rupert (Lord) Redesdale, my PA Vanessa Haines, and Shirley Williams. The idea was completely to encircle the place where the G8 leaders were having their meeting in a symbolic chain of debt - all pretty impressive. It worked, and afterwards, we all went to various venues for speeches and discussions. The organiser, economist Ann Pettifor, was a woman with amazing energy who never took 'no' for an answer. Fun it was too to walk through Birmingham Bullring and see Shirley greeted and hugged by total strangers. She is such a loved and loving person. She always responds to strangers in the same way she responds to everyone as if they are her close friends.

A series of meeting world figures followed that event. The Emperor and Empress of Japan came to Kew Gardens, but the encounter was even less memorable than meeting our Queen. I chatted to the Princess of Wales at the Royal Geographical Society during a conference on land mines and thought how completely ordinary she was and rather shy and self-effacing too. In the same period, it was over to the Wetlands in Barnes, for the newly developed Wild Fowl Trust there, in my constituency, and welcomed the Prince of Wales in a howling gale and heavy rain. His remarks were inaudible. A trip to New York to a conference on microcredit, which I had seen in action in Uganda, was financed by NGOs to celebrate the birthday of a truly great man, Muhammad Yunus, who founded the Grameen Bank in Bangladesh and started the whole microcredit movement. I loved New York, but they were having a fierce heatwave, and it was so cold in the conference centre that I had to buy a woolly to keep warm. Where is the sense in that America? That country is just civilisation and consumption gone mad. Another trip, as a UK representative to the OSCE, Organization for Security and Co-operation in Europe, Parliamentary Assembly in Copenhagen had to be endured as one of the UK representatives.

All these trips were followed by a Buckingham Palace garden party: a treat for Keith it was supposed to be, but unfortunately, he had an attack of diarrhoea, and after long hikes through the garden, trying to find a royal loo, we beat it back home. Being now a veteran of many garden parties, I can tell envious readers that apart from the exquisite cucumber sandwiches and tiny, delicious cakes, they are notable only for the funny hats worn by males and females and the fact that unless so honoured as to be chosen by flunkeys to shake hands with the Queen – must have gloves in case, says the protocol – you need binoculars to see her.

The soirée for MPs was much better value. My constituency workers were, quite rightly, beginning to wonder what exactly an MP was for as I headed for Venice and Florence for a breast cancer conference in my capacity as co-Chair of the All-Party Group for Breast Cancer. I had been delegated to speak on the group's behalf because of my previous life as a doctor. I had helped set up the first breast and cervical screening services in my health authority years before, so I did know a little about the subject. The final trip that year was back to a now freezing USA with the Select Committee for International Development to visit the UN and various aid-related organisations in the States. This time I visited Washington, the capital of the American Empire, and wondered at the massive buildings and awesome feel of the place like the minion I am, a citizen of what is soon to become the obedient province of the USA?

Constituency work is the work not appreciated by commentators who only see the performance of an MP in terms of attendance at debates, voting and the all-important media performances. I loved the parliamentary work and became a junkie on International Development. I was lucky too that because there were so few women MPs, especially in the two opposition parties, that I got a lot of media work. Question Time appearances are to die for, and I loved them. I appeared once or twice a season and on its radio sister programme Any Questions. It didn't make me very popular with male colleagues who felt the women got a better deal than them, just for once.

Constituency work is a combination of being like the Mayor and being a social worker. I often found myself at the same function as the Mayor. Every local event produces an invitation, and woe betides the MP who doesn't turn up. Many of them are extremely enjoyable, especially concerts, which are of a very high standard in Richmond and Kingston, and performances of all kinds. Many is the time, though, that a constituent has said, 'Wonderful to see you here relaxing, instead of working.' I am sad to say that I was often so tired that I would have preferred to be really relaxing in old clothes in front of the TV, which always did and does, send me to sleep very quickly. MPs have so little time to watch TV because evenings are spent in the House, so most start the day with the Today programme and end it with Newsnight, if back in time. My chief form of relaxation and creativity, if a speech was in the offing, was to get up with the lark and iron. I love ironing. Is it making the rough places smooth that appeals to me? I don't know, but it always allows me complete space to think and sort out problems.

Constituents' problems and sorting them out with the help of my staff was my least favourite activity. I was so fortunate to have as my caseworker and researcher in Richmond, one Serena Hennessy, who, besides being a local councillor, had worked as a journalist in her early years. She had an intimate knowledge of Richmond, warts and all. Best of all, she was blessed with a great sense of humour which made Friday sing along. The week always ended with 'surgeries' on Friday afternoons and Saturday mornings, and I did not enjoy it. Some MPs seem to love the feeling of power to help people, but I had been doing it all my life in GP surgeries and clinics, and it was no great novelty. Besides, the people who come to MPs' surgeries have often been everywhere else first, without satisfaction, and expect their MP to move the mountain that no one else could move. The most difficult to help and often the angriest are the mentally ill. I got a lot of these poor people, I suppose because of my medical background, but all MPs wrestle with these cases. Nigel Jones, when Liberal MP for Cheltenham had his assistant hacked to death in front of his eyes whilst trying to help a constituent, so there is apprehension from the staff in an MP's office if not from the MP herself. More recently, Jo Cox MP, mother of two small children, was killed when entering a building for a meeting in her own constituency. It is why threats and abuse are taken so much more seriously nowadays. The worst I had was a constituent who, if I was not there, would stand outside the premises screaming abuse about my staff and me until she either got tired or was removed by the police. I used to call my Friday surgery the Alternative Mental Health Out-Patient Department and was in close touch with the local mental health unit as a result. So much of the problem is lack of supervision of these poor souls from overworked and too few community staff. 'Care in the Community', much heralded by Mrs Thatcher, has become 'Neglect in the Neighbourhood', and the MP for the area is often on the receiving end.

One small constituent came up to town after an invitation from the Prime minister. Tony Blair, still fresh to the job and still engaging people, had asked MPs to select from their constituency a child who had had an unfortunate experience and had had to show great courage. The Richmond and North Kingston schools were asked to nominate children, and one child was finally selected to visit 10 Downing Street and have tea with Cherie Blair afterwards. My constituent was an 8-year-old boy whose mother had died following a long illness. We were greeted at the famous door by a policeman and, after a tour which included the chance to sit at the Cabinet table, tea was taken, and Cherie managed to speak to every child. Tony Blair himself then appeared and talked football with my guest after shaking his hand. The young boy vowed never to wash that hand again. The Blairs were such refreshing, powerful figures in those early years. Monkeys and backsides again spring to mind. How are the mighty fallen?

The dominant work for me during 1998 was monitoring the terrible famine which had southern Sudan in its grip. All through the year, there were worsening pictures on our TV screens of starving children and exhausted adults struggling to get to feeding centres. The Select Committee called an inquiry into what was going on and how, less than a decade from the Ethiopian famine, the world still seemed unprepared to cope. I remember how, during the time of the famine in Ethiopia, Bob Geldof inspired a generation about

Third World suffering. My lovely eldest son even went to midnight mass that Christmas, rockabilly hairstyle and all, and was congratulated by our parish priest for being young and concerned. He has remained concerned and interested and still is my greatest critic. I often bounce an idea off him first. I reflected during one committee session that the Ancient Egyptians had contingency plans for years of famine, and I could not understand why we do not have the modern equivalent of Pharaoh's granaries, stocked and ready to open in the lean years. Whether the international community had been distracted by the war in the Balkans during this time, I don't know, but I resolved to go and see for myself what was going on in Sudan.

Before I could go, the most important event in our family life was getting closer. I was asked to stand in for our Foreign Affairs Shadow Minister, Menzies (Ming) Campbell, and speak in a debate on the Middle East peace process, which was going nowhere. I had not been much involved at that time because, fortunately for the Palestinians, they were not a development issue then. I had remembered during my childhood having the creation of the state of Israel explained to me and praying for its future at church. As the details of the holocaust gradually filtered through to us all, it became the decent and loving thing to do. The Jews must have a safe place, and what better than their historical lands in Palestine? I thought of Gharda Karmi's story, my colleague in Ealing, but it was dismissed from my mind at that time.

My speech as Ming's deputy was duly prepared, with the help of the team researcher, and as I was waiting to speak, a message was passed to me from the Whips' Office. My son-in-law had telephoned to say that my daughter Mary was in labour and doing well in Kingston Hospital. I managed my speech and even looked forward to a more peaceful future for my first grandchild forging his way into the world. He would be in Hansard, although I didn't know he was a 'he' then, of course.

It was a curious feeling, pacing up and down Kingston Hill with Keith after being dismissed by Mary, who was having a long hard labour and preferred not to be watched by a crowd. Classic, gritty Mary. We had a pub meal amongst my constituents and went home to wait for the news of the baby's safe arrival and the celebrations that followed. Good to be back in the family circle for a while to enjoy the new arrival.

Chapter 13: The Poorest People on Earth

The enjoyment of our first grandchild and family life did not last for long. The East Africa officer for Christian Aid happened to be an old friend of my eldest son David and used to come to our house after school. He heard that I wanted to go to Sudan, so arrangements were made for him and the policy officer at Christian Aid to accompany me to southern Sudan if the Sudanese government would let us in. It was decided that we would go via Kenya, and the date was set for late January when I had done a bit of grandmothering. So it was that mischievous little Dan Collison, a frequenter of our house from the age of five to eleven, who I used to sometimes wait for in the school playground and see safely across roads, was to be my guide and guardian in southern Sudan, famine-stricken and in the grip of a decades-long civil war, with no hotels to stay in or parliamentary clerks to take care of me.

I was met at Heathrow by the policy officer, a curious, quiet man who knew an amazing amount about Africa. He was to become famous in my eyes for being able to drink huge amounts of water from a communal bottle without it touching his lips at all. He just poured it down. He also scorned insect repellents and anti-malarial drugs, preferring to flick a towel around himself at all times when outside. I was horrified at how nonchalant many of the aid workers are about malaria. I was obsessed with the fight against mosquitoes and their deadly cargo. My bedtime routine had to be seen to be believed as I covered my bed with a mozzie net, then sprayed it with Deet or whatever, then retired to lavatory or corridor whilst it settled, then climbed into bed through a tiny tunnel of net, fixed down on the inside by my torch, water bottle and book. Laugh, you may, but the only time the routine was wrecked was in Colombia, which I will come to later. Apart from that sad country, in ten years, I have only ever had mosquito bites in Europe. We flew overnight to Nairobi, which is very easy because it is 'down' the map, so you don't get jet lag, and I have short legs, so I don't get leg cramp either. Many are the times I have moved from coveted aisle seats to allow leggy colleagues a bit of room to stretch. I am designed for economy class. Nairobi had not changed from the previous year, but the hotel was not the Safari grandeur we had experienced on the Select Committee trip. It was an old hotel, much frequented by aid workers and extremely pleasant. The rooms were simple and overlooked gardens dripping with bougainvillaea. Dinner was taken in a large open dining area leading out to lawns and trees. I imagined that this trip would be OK after all in the comfort stakes. I had been told that accommodation would be basic or less and this was a very pleasant surprise.

We had a briefing over dinner on the situation as we would find it. We were going up to Bahr el Ghazal, which was just recovering from the worst of the famine but was still in the throes of civil war. It had just had the annual flooding from the waters of rivers joining up to form the White Nile as it flows into northern Sudan to join with the Blue Nile in Khartoum. We were warned that although some roads were passable, there were hardly any roads anyway, so tracks and walking would be our main means of getting about. The people were still on the move and not planting or growing crops because of the risk of raids, either from rebel (their own) troops or the dreaded Muraleen, who were Arab nomads from the north, encouraged by the government of Sudan to move south and rape, pillage and burn, a familiar story after recent events in Darfur. Aid was being dropped by the World Food Program on the area, most of it surplus grain from American farmers. A pretty depressing picture was painted all around.

It was in my room that night that I had an unexpected phone call from my head of office back in Richmond, Nick Carthew. Paddy Ashdown was standing down as leader of my party, the Liberal Democrats. Ten years as our leader was enough, and he felt the right time was now. It was very shocking news for everyone, but I felt particularly upset because there was nobody around who I could talk to, and the telephones were hopeless. So it all had to be tucked back into my head until I got back to the UK. I was here to concentrate on the problems of southern Sudan. I settled down after my mosquito routine to a good night's rest before real work started the next day.

On our first day, I was taken to a splendid house in the hills just above Nairobi, which I was told was the headquarters of the Sudan People's Liberation Movement/Army. It did not have its base in southern Sudan then, but thousands of miles away in Nairobi. There I was given apologies from John Garang, their leader, who was away (but not in Sudan) and was received by Commander Salva Kiir, then Deputy Leader, and Justin Yac, a much-respected elder of the Liberation Movement and representative of SPLM in East Africa. At that time, Salva Kiir always wore a full-coloured woollen cap on his head, which I did not see anyone else wearing anywhere in Sudan. He spoke very quietly and seemed not to have an ounce of enthusiasm or energy for his subject. Justin Yac was huge, not just tall like all the Dinka and Nuer people in the south, but wide too, with years of good food under his belt. I could not imagine he had ever been within sniffing distance of the famine. It seemed to me that the leaders had always been here, leading the civil war from afar. Something I found distasteful even before I saw the conditions in southern Sudan. The civil war had raged continuously for 20 years; over a million people were dead, countless numbers displaced, two major famines had occurred, and no solution was in sight.

From these two, I learned that the supply of arms to fight the war was no problem at all. A phone call to a broker in Europe or the UK meant that disused arms from the post-communist Eastern Bloc would be sent in via two or three other countries, such as Mozambique, Zambia, Zimbabwe or Angola. Libya had helped them, and Ethiopia had helped in the past. It was my first introduction to arms brokering which does so much damage in the world, and I was glad when I was put on the committee stage of the Export Control Bill dealing with such matters later on that year. Africa was, and still is, awash with arms, and we never seem to come to terms with it. Arms brokers are a scurrilous bunch in my eyes, trading as they do in human misery. They still operate under the noses of western governments, who seem to turn a blind eye.

Salva Kiir and Justin Yac accepted no responsibility for events and complained of the government of Sudan, who sent the Muraleen to torment the people without admitting any misdeeds by the rebel armies also committing crimes against civilians. As in Darfur later, one of the main problems was that the rebels split into two groups, and a key leader like Riek Machar changed sides several times. All this is done in the interests of the men concerned and has nothing to do with the poor civilians' needs, the elderly and women and children. Justin Yac wanted two separate countries but said the government of Sudan would never let this happen because of newly found oil reserves and the desire of the government to spread Islam and gain total control of the Nile. John Garang, he said, was wrong to want a secular, united Sudan, even as an interim measure. Wherever I went during the trip, I heard similar old men calling for the same things whilst quietly supporting one faction or other of the rebel groups. They were united on one thing only, which was that it was all the fault of Great Britain and that we should come back and sort out Sudan. Flattering, maybe, but I've never heard it suggested outside Sudan. The recently discovered oil in the area straddling the north and south of Sudan was a major factor, although dismissed by the people in the south who declared, 'The oil will never flow!'

I resolved to bear all this in mind when I got home because it was obvious that southern Sudan was stuck in the age-old cycle of poverty leading to unrest and civil war, which cause even greater poverty and unrest. A political and support solution was found eventually, forming two nations of Sudan and South Sudan, with South Sudan controlling the oil and Sudan receiving huge revenue from transporting it via a pipeline to Port Sudan for export. The war in South Sudan between Nuer and Dinka still festers, and the people in neither country are much better off. The Christian Aid team and I were taken by small aircraft to a place called

Lokichoggio in northern Kenya. Looking out of the aircraft windows, we saw Mount Kenya and the wonderful open savannah dotted with those spreading flat-topped trees. We could easily see wildlife from the plane because they fly fairly low. To me, these trips in small aircraft are the nearest thing to flying under your own steam. It is so exhilarating compared with the 'canned' feeling you get in big aircraft. Known as 'Loki' for short, this was the nerve centre and base for the mighty 'Operation Lifeline Sudan', which had been set up by the UN and the World Food Programme to feed the people during the famine. It was a moving scene. Pharaoh's Granary! Hundreds of sacks of wheat stored in hangers and piled up along the runway, where several old Hercules aircraft stood ready to be loaded. They operated 100 sorties a day, dropping food on 100 different places in the area. There were no roads, so this was the only way to get aid in. There was no guarantee that the people would reach the food before one or other armed group, but I was told this is a risk they have to take.

The pleasant climate of Nairobi had been replaced by a windy blistering heat with dust blown around everywhere. I jammed my hat on my head and a thin cotton scarf around my mouth, and we walked towards the compound. Operation Lifeline Sudan, Lokichoggio, was straight out of M*A*S*H, that TV series set in the Korean War. Neatly laid out roads, low huts with iron roofs and the odd tent here and there housed 360 personnel, who hailed from the UN, WFP (the World Food Program) and NGOs. All the NGOs seemed to be there, all competing with each other for the smartest office. I began to wonder again about where the donated money went. Whilst I was wondering, I was introduced to a great character, Achul, who was to accompany us into Bahr el Ghazal the next day. He asked me to open the new office of SUDAID, a local partner of Christian Aid in Sudan. It bore the proud banner outside 'SUDAID OFFICE donated by DFID UK'. I duly cut the pink ribbon, said a few words, and wondered what Clare Short would say when I reported back. Offices before aid was my first impression of Loki. We were allocated very respectable huts belonging to aid workers who had gone on leave and directed to where the showers and latrines were, also very adequate, even if quite a walk away – and needing shoes in case of *snakes,* I was told. The mess was another revelation, with a huge choice of food and drink. Poignant, when we considered that outside the gates of the compound were villages full of emaciated people with nothing to eat. Some of them were gathered around the gates almost permanently in case a morsel of food was dropped by people going in and out of the camp.

That evening we mustered for a security briefing. The Commander of the camp strode in, looking a bit like Hawkeye in M*A*S*H, and told us what to expect over the next twelve hours in that official military speak the Americans are so good at. The Lord's Resistance Army was very active again on the Uganda/Kenya border. This despicable group raids villages at night and captures children who are taken away to fight or be the soldiers' sex slaves. It was the stuff of nightmares.

The Government of Sudan were bombing the area. The Muraleen, forerunners of the Janjaweed of Darfur fame, were coming down on the train to Wau bringing supplies to the government forces and were allowed to rape and pillage as much as they liked on the way. The train travels very slowly, so the Muraleen were able to do their dirty work and then return to the train for a lift to the next populated area. Both the Muraleen and the Janjaweed come from roaming cattle herders who were becoming more and more impoverished as pasture dried up and were happy to move south onto other lands. There always was a tension between them and their pastoralist cousins in the south who stayed put. These Muraleen, however, were deadly.

Kerambino, one of the rebel leaders, was reported to be regrouping his troops near Turalei, where we were going the next day. Cattle rustling, rape and pillage were continuing as it has done for generations, my colleagues added, both between the Arabs in the north and the animists in the south and between the various tribes,

Nuer and Dinka most notably. A lawless land. The briefing ended with a click of the heels, and Hawkeye marched out. I slept fitfully that night with my torch under my pillow. Thankfully I met no snakes on my way to the showers.

We started early the following day and went back to the airstrip, where the Hercules was already being loaded with the day's food drop. The situation then had improved a little, but there was still very little food around. The World Food Programme (WFP) people take wild foods into account too, when they assess the situation, and I was to realise how crucial berries and seeds could be to starving people. The vegetation is stripped of anything edible. Fish are sometimes caught, but only in the rainy season. This land alternates between flooding and drought. The basic nutritional need is around 2000 calories a day for people doing hard physical activity all day. We consume that sort of amount when we go on a diet! Last year over 50 per cent of the population had been below this level, but this year only 20 per cent. With no prospects of growing any food because of the constant raids, this was still a very precarious position.

I also learned that although no one knew whether AIDS had come to the area, southern Sudan is home to every disease known to man, and the population is sick and weak. Big campaigns had been waged against polio, measles and vitamin deficiency, but the main scourge was malaria, with 100,000 cases reported every year. Mosquito nets and medicines are unheard of here. Terrible to reflect that under the British administration, there had been health care and schools and a proper administration, even it is was by someone else. The civil war had destroyed everything. The need for peace was the greatest 'need' of all. No wonder the old men wanted the British back!

We landed on a small bumpy airstrip that was surrounded by grizzled trees and bush—dry, hot, unwelcoming. The aircraft was immediately surrounded by extremely tall Dinka men, some in long white robes and carrying staffs, but many in any old T-shirt and shorts. I saw one Manchester United shirt amongst the melee. I was later to learn that, as in Uganda and Kenya, football teams are an international language, even if the only English spoken is the name of their favourite team. Most of them were carrying old cans for any kerosene the pilot could spare. We then trudged through the heat for about half an hour, followed silently by this motley crew and trying to listen to Stephen Myong, the Acting DC for Twic County, which was the name of this part of Bahr el Ghazal.

We were taken to the compound where we were to spend two nights which, we were told, was the home of Justin Yac's mother. My expectations rose. Surely the mother of the great man living a life of Riley in Nairobi must be well cared for. Well, she was, by Twic County standards. The compound was surrounded by a rough wooden stockade with gates that were closed at night. Inside was a group of about six dark, dirty, circular huts with straw roofs and a latrine, fondly known to us forevermore as the long drop, sited at the edge of the compound. The whole area was only a diameter of about 20 or 30 yards.

I wondered which hut I would get and how on earth I would survive the night, but before I could ask, we were taken in procession to meet the great matriarch of the Yac family. She was a truly lovely woman, as old as time and very wizened, but with an energy and sparkle that seemed to say she would survive anything. We thanked her, and I presented her with a House of Commons trinket, very acceptable, I was told, if entirely inappropriate. We were always told to take small gifts wherever we went.

We were then whisked away for another briefing under a nearby tree from the Acting District Commissioner. The main messages were what became depressingly familiar over the next two days. The war had caused great displacement, and people could not grow any food. Even if they had salvaged some seed, the crop would be destroyed in the next raid, and they were reliant on food aid. The Government of Sudan were not interested because the southern Sudanese are animists or Christians (thanks to those missionaries) and therefore were infidels. Oh, why did you have to interfere Albert Schweitzer and your ilk? The cattle had been driven away or lost, and there was no milk for the children. The UK is responsible because we left Sudan too quickly with Egypt in charge in the north, and it was *our* responsibility to sort it out.

The evening started with an invitation to take a shower. This consisted of a bucket full of river water which was hauled up into a tree a little way away, but certainly no privacy. I watched as an English woman, who had joined us in the compound, had her shower. She soaped herself with her own bar of soap which she told me was her little 'luxury' and then untied the bucket, and the water lashed over her, and she was clean. She put her clothes back on and rejoined the group. I found this performance very strange. Women in southern Sudan are well covered up and almost invisible until the men want food. They certainly showed little of themselves when I was there, except to show me when asked the endless round of hard labour they performed for the men. Yet this western woman was there with a scanty vest and shorts, wearing only rubber flip flop shoes and displaying an enormous amount of pale brown, leathery, skinny body and breasts. I felt embarrassed for her, but she was untroubled. She worked for an NGO but had made Sudan her home and had been here for years. I have to say that the men took little notice of her either, but I found the whole evening uncomfortable. I was watching this skinny vision in case she suddenly decided to entertain us more. I made do with a wash and declined the striptease behind the tree!

We all sat around a rough table in the compound and ate the special meal for the visitors from England. The first course was okra soup which was watery and tasted like vomit. We forced it down with sorghum wheat bread which is flat and unleavened and is very rough and scratchy. I helped make it the next morning when the women showed me how to hand grind the wheat into rough flour and then bake it on hot stones. We were truly blessed to get the next course, which was spiny fish that someone had caught that day. Not very appetising, but it had taken the boys all day to catch enough for the feast. That was it, all washed down with our own supply of water. I had to remind myself that this was the headmen's compound, and this was a huge feast by the standards of southern Sudan in recent months.

As darkness fell, I realised that the boys were putting up one-person tents for us – we were not going to sleep in those huts after all. I don't think anyone did except Grandmother Yac. The huts were for storage when they had anything to store. The people slept on the ground outside to guard their precious possessions. I crawled through the tent flap, taking care not to let in the dreaded mosquitoes, unrolled my mat and settled for the night. I arranged my bag, kissed goodnight the photograph of my new grandson and hoped he would give my daughter and her husband a quiet night. He seldom did. He was a very feisty baby. I drifted into sleep to the sound of drums beating their rhythm across Bahr el Ghazal. I had been warned that they would continue because although we could not interpret the messages, they were relating the progress of the famous train full of Muraleen and whether or not it had got to a stopping point. I was told later, back in Kew, by an African performer, that African drums were the first mobile phones! They transmit urgent messages very efficiently, as did the beacon fires of mediaeval England. No time for gossip, though.

Halfway through the night, I needed the lavatory. I had kept well hydrated, and I congratulated myself before realising that I wasn't in Nairobi or even in the compound at Lokichoggio, but in the middle of Sudan under the stars, and the 'long drop' toilet was at the far side of the compound. I had used it during the day and not been very happy. It had a fence for privacy, and the 'seat' consisted of a raised circle of clay. The drop was long, stinking and full of flies which rose up to greet you as you peed, women always at a disadvantage because we have to sit or squat and cannot just hose down the flies like the men. It was the most awful thing for a person passionate about the contribution Victorian sewage engineers had made to our society. Their contribution was greater than that of physicians and surgeons to the health of the population. Life for me without a flushing loo is a misery to be borne only occasionally. That day, after one visit, I had resolved to walk away from the compound and find a bush, rather as one does in the European countryside when taken short. The flies were just too much. Anyway, it was getting urgent, and I reckoned the flies would not be around in the night air, which had become quite cold. In any case, everyone, people, cows, dogs alike, were locked in the compound for the night.

I crawled out of my tent and surveyed the scene. There was no moon that night, and although the stars were magnificent, they did not provide much light. I groped as best as I could towards the compound periphery in the direction of the long drop, which I found fly-free to my delight, and set off back to my tent. But somehow, I made off in the wrong direction. I first bumped into a large furry object which turned out to have large horns. The cow must have been as amazed as I was to find a human being nearly kissing her in the middle of the night. She made a bit of a mooing sound which set the dogs off. Nobody came to my rescue. Were they asleep, I wondered, or just trembling in their tents and huts, thinking the drums were wrong and the Muraleen were upon us? I shushed the dogs, who, for some reason, fell quiet again. Luckily I realised that I was by the rough table we had used for supper earlier, and I knew my tent was just down to the right of that. I stumbled thankfully into it, pausing for a moment to stargaze.

I love the stars. Now I was comfortable and safely back near my tent; I spent a few minutes gazing upwards. I have never seen the stars better anywhere than in Africa. You can almost touch them. I think I remember seeing Orion up there. I look for him everywhere I go, and sometimes I am lucky, and it's the right time. I like to think he protects me from all ills in a quaint, primitive sort of way. He was certainly on guard that night. I could have raised the whole village. No one had heard me when I told my tale the next morning, but I guess they might have been being tactful.

I woke up wondering where on earth I was. It was cold, so I had wrapped up in my mosquito net during the night after my trip of terror to the long drop. I lay there half-awake pondering and listening to Lillibulero on a very crackly radio. I gradually realised where I was and that someone had an old radio and was listening to the World Service in the middle of the countryside in southern Sudan. I later found out that it was William, one of the elders, who listened every morning when he had batteries, and so was the sage on world affairs for his area.

The World Service should be one of the treasures in the UK. It is revered in Africa and is often the only communication out in the bush. It was great to hear that tune, and I thought of telling the World Service guys at the BBC when I got back. I suppose mobile phones have now taken over the role of William's old radio – if there is any network in South Sudan.

Lying there, now fully awake, I decided that a solution had to be found to my weak bladder at night and the fear of the long drop. My practical and much-travelled eldest son had given me two incredibly useful things for my first 'rough' trip – he disregards ones organised by parliament as being luxury tours. A soft neck pillow was one such present, much used in light aircraft and bumpy Land Rovers lurching through the bush. The other present was a small knife, very sharp. That night, after we had all retired, I switched on my torch and cut an empty plastic bottle in two. With the top inverted in the bottom, I had made a super potty which I could then crouch over when nature called. It worked that night and subsequently. In the morning, I slung its contents down the long drop and rinsed it out with my precious water. I was very proud of myself, although I often wonder if any of the Dinka in our compound saw my shadowy figure through my tent walls, doing strange things and making strange sounds. They might have thought it was some curious religious rite or English ritual. If they did, they never said.

Whilst staying with Mrs Yac senior, we undertook to meet with the local people to hear their concerns and say what we were doing in

Twic County. We walked to a large tree one day, which was the muster point for the meeting. It took about an hour to walk there, but when we arrived, there were hundreds of men, women and children, many of whom had walked for several days to the meeting to see and hear what had been billed (by the drums) as a MEMBER OF THE BRITISH PARLIAMENT. I was humbled.

The people in southern Sudan blamed the British for their problems. We should not have left when we did. They listen to the tales of the elders of how the British ruled southern Sudan and how the children went to school and the sick received health care. Halcyon days they were, in their collective memory. We had to leave Sudan, the administration of which had been shared with Egyptians, as a result of the Marshall Plan. This was America's aid package for Europe after the Second World War, which had been agreed, on the condition that European nations gave up their colonies. A few survived without war, but southern Sudan and the government in Khartoum, run by the Arab inheritors of the Egyptian rule, had been at war ever since. Apart from a relatively quiet ten years in the middle, there had been a civil war in Sudan, unreported in the west for forty years, punctuated by terrible famines. Millions had died, and millions more had been displaced to the north or abroad as refugees. The two great famines had hit the headlines, the most recent one being the reason for this trip.

I was introduced, and a silent crowd with solemn faces hung on my every word. Even the children were silent. They were all stick thin but sat relaxed and elegant under the tree. The Dinka and Nuer of southern Sudan are extremely tall, very fine-featured, and jet, jet black. Is this all as a result of natural selection to cope with the severe droughts interspersed with flooding from the Nile every year and relentless hot sun? Could this be Darwin's Theory in action I pondered?

I talked of the assessments we were making and how I wanted to listen to what they had to say so that I could tell my government what their needs were. It all sounded so trite. What could I do to lift these people out of the most abject poverty I had ever seen in my life? They had nothing, and I mean nothing. Many had had their animals stolen and their homes burned down. They were back to living as hunter-gatherers, except there was little left to hunt apart from a few spiny fish in the wet season. I had noticed few birds in the area, kites mainly: that's because they had all flown away from the devastation that was Bahr el Ghazal in 1999. Only Justin Yac's mother and her family seemed to have escaped, with a few animals and enough wood to rebuild the stockade, but live on, they did. The human spirit is extraordinary.

My speech was followed by a long rant from a lovely but very voluble old man called William, of World Service radio fame, who had been to university in the UK long ago. He had come back to his people to share their pain. He exhorted them to stop the inter-tribal fighting which was going on, preventing a united front from being formed to fight the north or to parley for peace. This I learned is the curse of Sudan. Rebel groups form along tribal lines and fight each other as well as the enemy. Every man seems to think that the possession of a gun means success and riches, like the government in the north. This was well demonstrated by another speech that afternoon given by a young man in half of a very smart uniform, with a jaunty Sudan People's Liberation Army beret on. He waved a Kalashnikov and told the enthralled crowd that only *he* could protect them because he had a gun and men with guns are the powerful ones. The little boys inched closer to their hero figure, hoping no doubt to grow up one day to be a soldier with a fine gun. Once again, poverty breeds war, breeds poverty, breeds war. This relentless cycle is so depressing.

I was asked again to speak and conclude the meeting, which had lasted over three hours – they do not expect less when they walk so long and so far for the great event. I explained how we were hoping to get more help into the area, but most of all, to pursue the then embryonic peace process. Everything had to be translated from English into Nuer and Dinka, so I was never quite sure where we had got to. I then presented the headmen with House of

Commons pens, which I had been told would be very acceptable. It seemed to me the daftest thing ever when no one had any paper to write on. It was a bit like handing out 'Crackerjack' pencils on the English children's TV programme my kids used to watch. Nevertheless, they were accepted graciously and displayed proudly to the crowd. These little episodes make me feel so ashamed.

One of the needs expressed that afternoon I had already been told about by Dan Collison. In the flood season, the men fish with homemade spears, and it's a long and laborious process. It had occurred to one of the NGO lads that fishing lines with multiple hooks might be easier for them, and they were longing to try. Requests to DFID had brought the incredible response that if they strayed from traditional methods of fishing, they might run out of fish! I wondered if the dodo who gave that response had ever been out of Whitehall. On my return, I made sure the message got through, and the people got some fishing lines eventually.

The other request I was unable to satisfy. When people are living in war, there is no education. This is terrible for the women because they can never get on with their mountainous chores without all the children being with them. It also meant that after forty years, there were two generations in southern Sudan who were illiterate and innumerate. I spent a good deal of effort on my return trying to get DFID to fund the basics for education in southern Sudan. It is not as if vast resources are needed: a large tree, of which there were still a few remaining in most villages; some slates; and chalk and a blackboard. A man who had been a teacher at some stage told me that the children are very keen to learn. The simple tools he needed could be taken away with the villagers if they were attacked. The villages were constantly under attack, but they always tried to carry the basics into hiding – simple cooking utensils were the only thing they seemed to possess. DFID would have none of it. You cannot fund 'education' in conflict zones; that was that. Never mind if the conflict came and went over years – some areas might be peaceful for months on end. So many children with nothing to do except hope to grow big enough to hold a gun and be a soldier, which was the only ambition they could have if they wanted food and clothing.

Later that afternoon, I asked to meet with the women alone. A pretty radical request, it seemed. The women in southern Sudan were the property of the men, and polygamy was quite common in this Christian/animist society. Women were not talked to because they had no opinions and knew nothing. So what could I possibly mean? Wanting to talk to the women indeed! I persisted in my nicest 'lady doctor understands' mode. I just wanted to gossip and find out what they did when it was too dark to work, and the men were gathered around the fire for their important strategic chat. It was a revelation. Nine women from the area gathered under a tree. We were surrounded by the men all standing around at a distance. I beat them back out of earshot. Luckily they seemed quite amused. This mad English woman MP (token man) wanting to talk to women and not them. The women were worried about food and the shortage of animals, which were always taken by the Muraleen when they raided. Their main concern was that many of the women had stopped menstruating, and this was serious to them only because their men would get cross that they were not having babies. They were all malnourished, and I wondered whether this was a common feature amongst women after a famine. Girls who develop anorexia in the West also get amenorrhoea, so there could be a connection.

Another nugget of information was that girls marry as soon as they menstruate, which is around 15 years old – much later than our girls. Oh yes, and when they are menstruating, they are allowed only goats' milk to drink and no food, which means they are even more malnourished because all the goats had gone. This means more complications during pregnancy and childbirth and very poor maternal and child mortality figures. Try telling all this to the affluent middle classes of Richmond, I thought, not just thankful for safe delivery, but demanding exotica like water births and the same midwife all through their pregnancy (no midwives here) and that euphemism called 'natural childbirth'. The women in Sudan *all* have a natural childbirth. What wouldn't they give for any old midwife and a whiff of gas and air? Infections were common, and I think so was FGM, that awful practice that we were to investigate later on in parliament. Nobody would talk about these things, though, not even with the men absent. I did establish that syphilis and gonorrhoea were around, these being caused apparently by 'someone treading on the grave of a maternal uncle'.

The complaints then thundered on. Money does not exist out here, and they were lucky to have the clothes they stood up in and a shared cooking pot or two. Once again, I repeat, I never knew such poverty existed, but lie down and die they do not. The human spirit carries on. They look forward to the war ending, life returning, and most of all, for some food to give the children, of which there still seemed to be plenty, despite the worries about infertility. I asked them what they would like as a little present from me if I got it sent out from Nairobi as a thank you for their time and frankness with me. They requested a tea set! Dan explained to me that when the men have their (very important) meetings every day, whilst the women work, they drink tea or hot water if there are no tea leaves, out of little glass cups and a special flask. They always managed to save it from the raiders, and it had taken on mystic importance. The women longed for the same. I was able to send out exactly what they wanted a few months later with the next visit an NGO made to that area, and I love to think of them sitting under that tree with their *very* superior tea set, sipping their hot water from cups instead of sharing an old can. I hope it has survived. Before I left the village a couple of days later, I was presented with a rough brass bangle to wear to remember them – I still wear it often. It is made from the melted down bullet cartridges left behind by the militia, the only riches they have. I promised to wear it until there was a peace agreement, which there was briefly in 2004.

When we returned to Mrs Yac's compound that night, the young boys of the family asked to see our video camera. A thing from outer space! It had been loaned to me by BBC2 programme-makers and their presenter Shaun Ley, who did regular updates in those days on what our London MPs were up to, in a programme called 'Around Westminster'. I managed to get the picture of a lifetime which I proudly displayed in the members' photographic exhibition when I got back. A young impoverished Dinka boy was peering through our camera, a bit of high-tech equipment the like of which he could only dream about.

Every day in Sudan, just as it was getting light, breakfast was always water or 'tea', which did not resemble any tea I knew. It was certainly not good old builder's tea – I have never been a drinker of fancy teas. As honoured guests, we were also offered a 'Nice' biscuit from an ancient tin that must have been Mrs Yac's present from her son when he last visited. They were very soft and stale indeed but very welcome, as no one else ate anything until the evening meal in this god-forsaken place. There was nothing to eat, full stop. That morning we walked through the swamps to visit a family living rough in the bush after being raided some months before. The swamps were deep. I got more and more anxious as the water level reached mid-thigh, and for the last few yards, I was carried like a baby by 7ft tall Achul to stop it going up over my waist! A routine operation for him. I was thankful, having imagined snakes, or at the very least leeches attaching themselves to me. No such terrors occurred, thanks to our lofty Dinka colleagues.

The family we met on the far side of the swamp had been attacked in the evening by Arab militia, and most had run off into the bush. There followed a very confusing story from a young girl who had been tending goats when the attack occurred and had come back to find their huts torched and animals gone. She was captured then released by the 'Arabs' when she told them she was a Kerumbimo commander's daughter – a local warlord. It reminded me of my childhood when I was confronted by rough kids in the Midlands. I would always say, 'My dad's a policeman,' and they would run away. Telling them my dad was a headteacher never occurred to me. Police officers were held in much greater reverence in those days. She was then recaptured and forced to watch whilst an uncle was tortured to death by being disembowelled and beaten. He would not say where the family had gone, and so he died. This poor girl had then wandered the swamps for days with the 'Arabs' and was given no food. She said she had not been raped, or if she had, she would not admit it because that would cast her out into the darkness for sure, even from her own family. Somehow she had escaped and got back to her family, but I do not think that even she knew how. Subsequently, this girl had been married off by her family for 70 head of cattle which had made them seriously rich again. Whether there would be enough grazing for those cows was the perennial problem in southern Sudan, where global warming is causing the desert to spread south and all tribes with it, in a desperate search for food. We went back through the swamps, blazing with water lilies and pink convolvulus and giant water snails.

That afternoon we visited a GOAL feeding station that had been set up during the famine and was still operating, of course. The guy in charge, Fergus, was Irish. He had a host of stories about the inappropriateness of some aid efforts. A consignment of clothes had come from Oxfam a few months before and was eagerly fallen upon by the local people, only a few of whom have the traditional white robes and turbans you used to see in the geography books. Most Dinka and Nuer here wore whatever came from Oxfam and other charities, and the children wore nothing. This largest consignment was obviously from a well-heeled part of the UK – Richmond? I wondered. The men fell on the brightly coloured ski-suits and salopettes that fell out of the bags and put them on with great delight. Seven-foot-tall Dinka men in bright red and blue ski wear and the temperature around 45 degrees centigrade. They were delighted but took them off pretty quickly. Does anyone actually *think* before they send such nonsense? The best tale of all was the one about the 'free' students. The local Catholic bishop who was in overall charge of aid projects in this area had been offered four 'free' students, plus extra funding, by the US National Association of Protestant Salvation, which he had accepted readily and with an open mind because the need was so great. The students came and settled happily, teaching in the tiny village school. One day one of the children told Fergus that they had been taken to the river by the students, submerged, and apparently 'baptised' into an evangelist faith. The children were happy but a little confused. The confusion became greater when the local bishop, having consulted the Archbishop in Khartoum, was told to take the children back down to the river and re-baptise them into the Catholic faith. Oh, Western Christians, what did you do to these little ones? Fergus' comment was, 'What the hell will these kids think of us when, it seems, every time they see a white man, they get carted off to the fucking river and pushed under?'

We drank beer that night as the stars came out and pondered on such tales. I wondered what it would be like if when your husband dies, his brother, son, father or cousin takes you on as another wife. The generations become mixed up and confused, but I guess it's better than being alone, trying to survive in this hostile environment.

The next day we were up early once again and walked to the tiny airstrip to wait for our lift back to Lokichoggio. As the plane came in to land, men appeared out of the bush once again with big plastic cans to beg a little kerosene from the pilot, who seemed happy to oblige. It was a happy scene, with most of the people around gathered to bid farewell to this strange, plump little MP from the UK. It was the first time anyone had stayed longer than a day in the war/famine zones. Other MPs had come with cameras, photographed the starving babies with their pot bellies and flies and flown out again. I could be a little bit pleased that I had lasted longer than that. We had a superb flight back over the swamps and bush of southern Sudan into northern Kenya and the base camp. We dined that night safari style in the commander's compound on obscene amounts of food. I know that aid workers must be looked after, but it was a stark contrast, not just to where I had just been, but to the starving Masai people outside the gates of the compound.

After a long 'wash-up' meeting with UNICEF and others, we decided on the priorities for 1999. The emergency food drops must continue, as wild foods were scarce, and little planting could take place because of the war. However, we resolved to push urgent seed supplies and tools for those areas which were quiet. Disease prevention by vaccination was continuing, but the need for education at its simplest level was urgent, and I promised to push this, with not much chance of success I feared. Roads needed to be built and landmines cleared, but there was no prospect of this until peace was brokered. 'Oh lovely peace, with plenty crowned' – the greatest prize of all.

On my return to the UK and parliament, Hylton Dawson, the Labour MP for Lancaster (who had a Sudanese Dinka man working in his office), and I founded the All-Party Parliamentary Group for Sudan. We not only visited Sudan again and again but got very embroiled in the peace process led by Senator John Danforth of the USA and ex-Ambassador Alan Goulty of the UK.

A fragile peace descended on southern Sudan in 2005, and I was able to take off my bangle! Sadly, by that time, a repeat performance war of rebels versus government-backed militia was raging in Darfur. Dan Collison, who had cared for me better than I ever cared for him as a child, got a bad attack of malaria on our way back to Nairobi, the price many of our aid workers pay for their concern.

Still fascinated by Sudan, Keith and I were contacted by Zeinab Badawi, the BBC World Service presenter, to ask if we could help with the personal project she had set up to ask the NHS to give up redundant medical and surgical equipment and help transport it to Sudan, where Omdurman Hospital was in an appalling state. Keith came with us during a parliamentary recess to assess the needs, which were everything, including beds and curtains. The patients lay on beds - if they were lucky to have one at all - with no coverings or privacy. Zeinab, with great charm and determination, managed to get a whole pantechnicon of equipment over to Port Sudan and have it transported to Omdurman. A haematologist was also part of the team trying to get a blood donation system established—no mean feat.

We also checked up on village women's services which we had seen and been horrified by. Villages seemed to have a key person who did deliveries – traditional 'birth attendants' they are called, or TBAs. We met one such who was very richly dressed and even had a Gucci handbag. Fees must have been high. We learned later that she also did the FGMs in that area, so she was on to a nice little earner. Sickening to think of it when she did not possess any equipment to measure blood pressure in her patients, a pretty basic requirement for anyone looking after pregnant women.

I have returned to Sudan on three subsequent occasions. The All-Party Group for Sudan went out to see what was happening in Darfur, and I stayed instead in Khartoum and went to Omdurman to see how our equipment had fitted in, brought with such effort from the NHS to Sudan. The director of the hospital warned me that I would get a shock and proudly showed me around a completely transformed hospital with shiny white walls and labs and decent wards for the patients. Apparently, when the government heard what Zeinab, with her high profile in the UK, had done, they had immediately released money for the hospital to be re-equipped.

It is a troubled region, but the UK government was very keen to help the Sudanese in the north and south separate into two countries. The arrangement did not last long because civil war and dreadful killings broke out in South Sudan between mainly Dinka and Nuer people, Salva Kiir and Riek Machar being the main protagonists. This stopped the flow of oil, and terrible fighting continued in Darfur, dealt with brutally by the Khartoum government. Poverty still reigns in most of South Sudan, and apart from a few rich business people, the same applies to Sudan. I wondered again whether the women would make a better job of it, but when you are very poor and cannot feed or clothe your children, the boys will get both if they join an army and start fighting. It is very depressing. As I write, the sanctions imposed by the west after the Khartoum government's actions in Darfur are gradually being lifted, and on a recent visit, the group saw some signs of optimism. A relatively peaceful civilian revolution led mainly by women has taken place. Omar al-Bashir, the deposed president of Sudan, is currently awaiting trial at the International Criminal Court and joint military and civilian government are in power. Dare we hope?

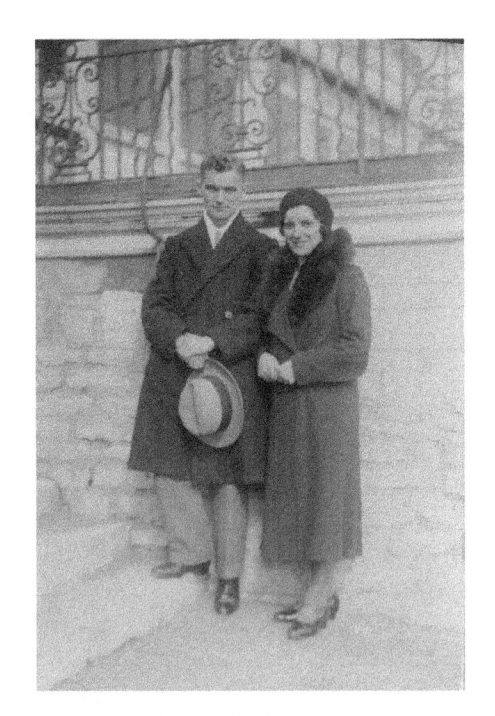

My parents on honeymoon

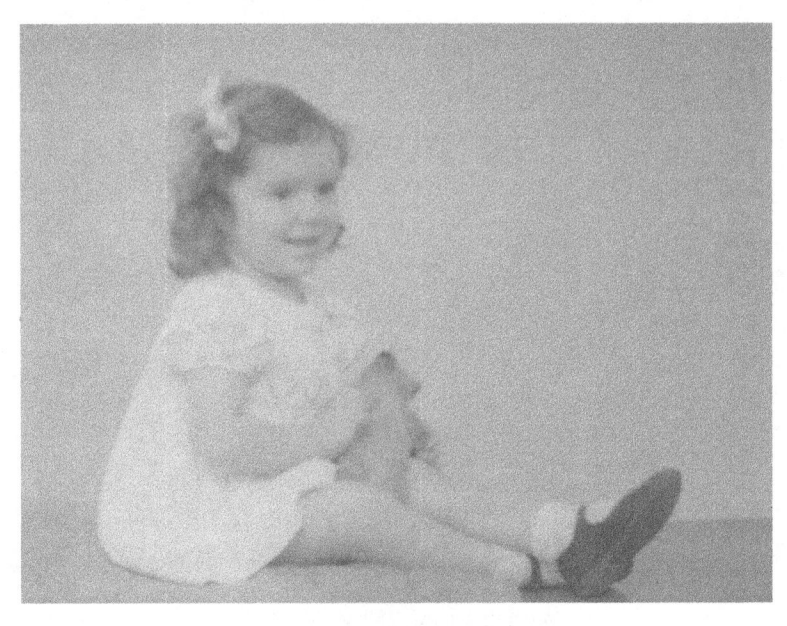

The author, age 3

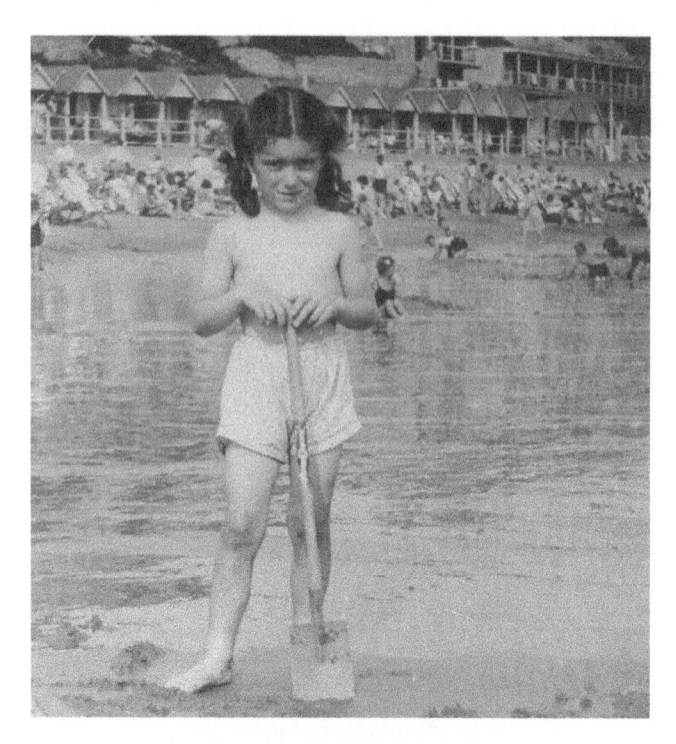

Age 7 on Bournemouth Beach

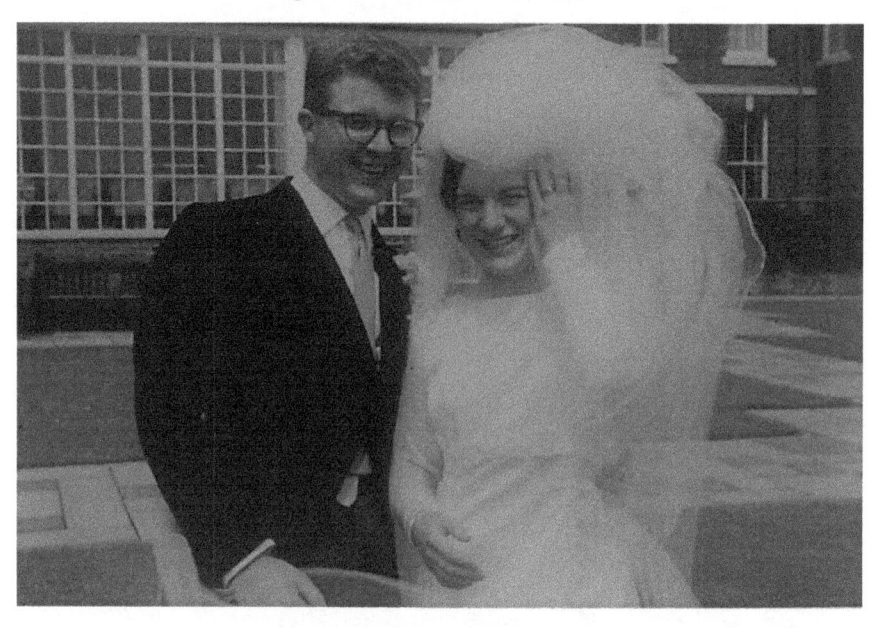

Wedding Day, 23rd May 1964

133

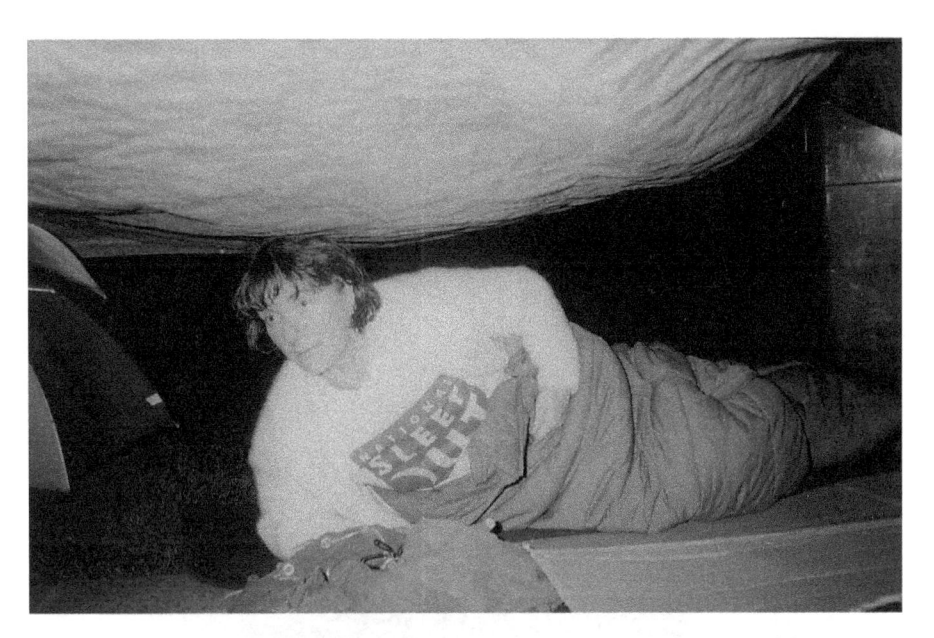

Campaign Against Sleeping Rough, Shene School Playing Fields

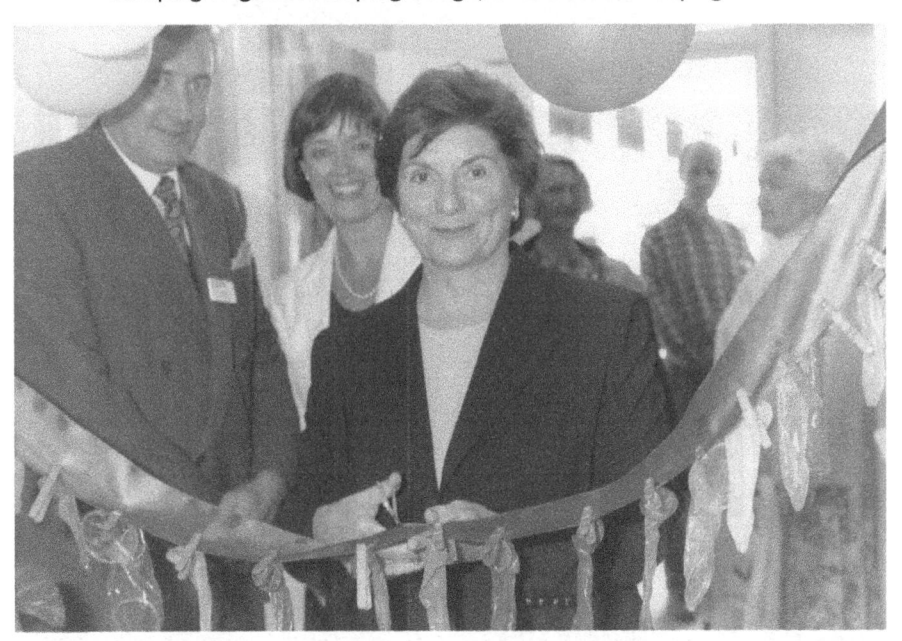

Opening the new Sexual & Reproductive Health Clinic at Kingston Hospital

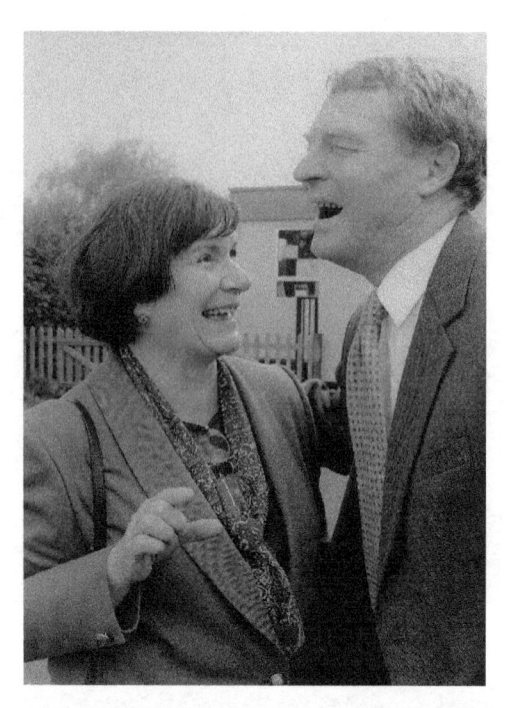

On the campaign trail with Paddy Ashdown

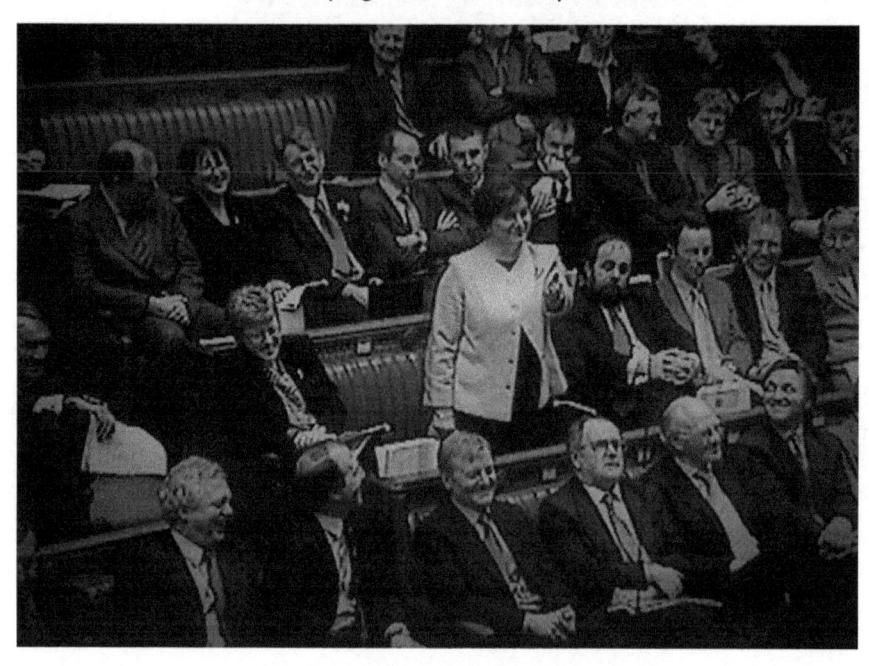

In the House of Commons

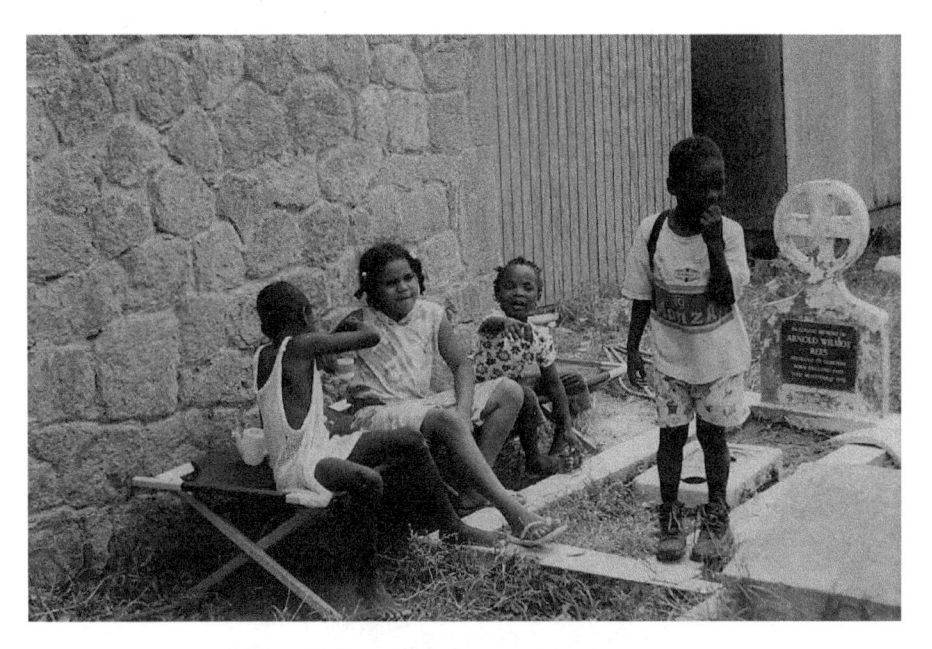

Children living in the graveyard in Montserrat

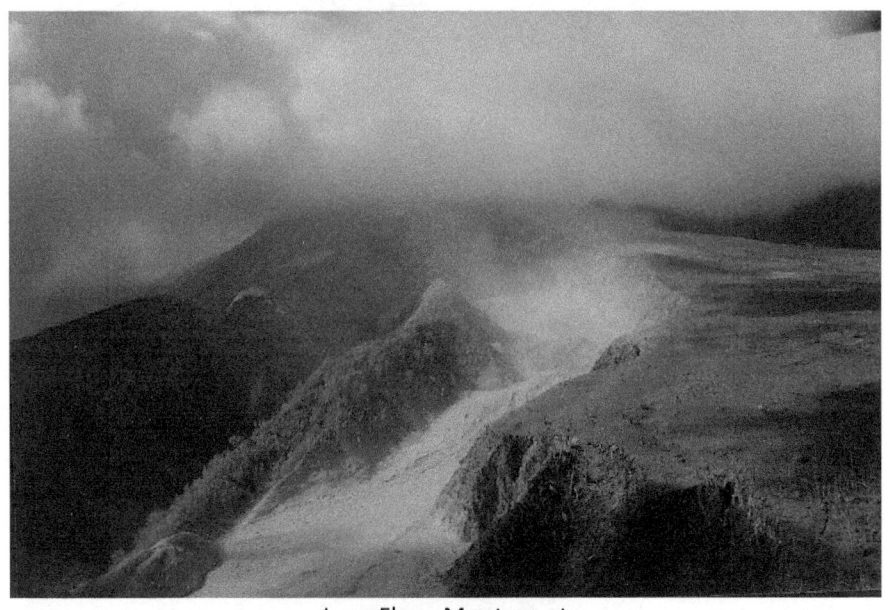

Lava Flow. Montserrat

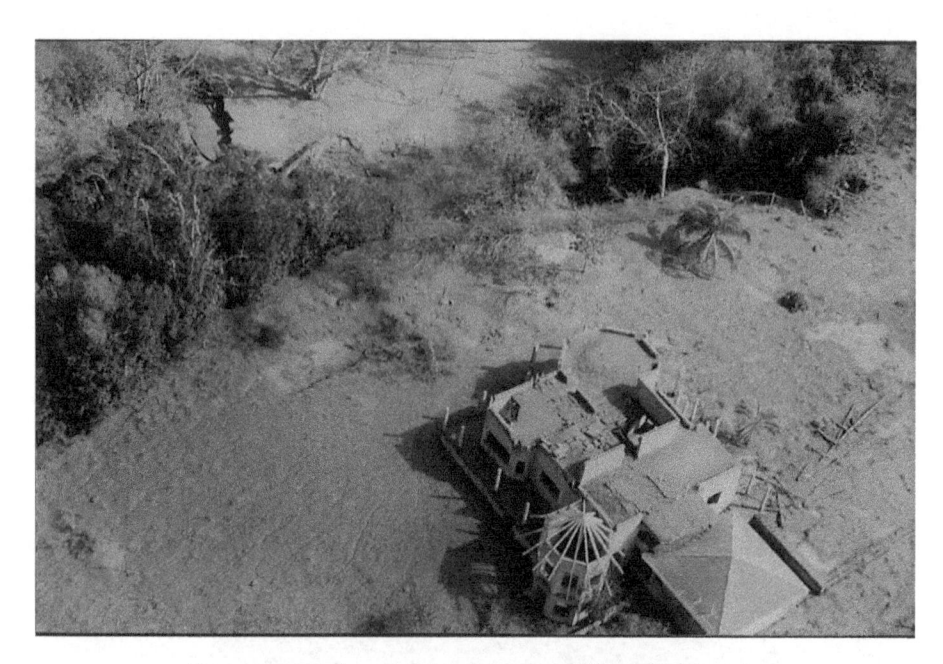

Government House, Montserrat, under volcanic ash

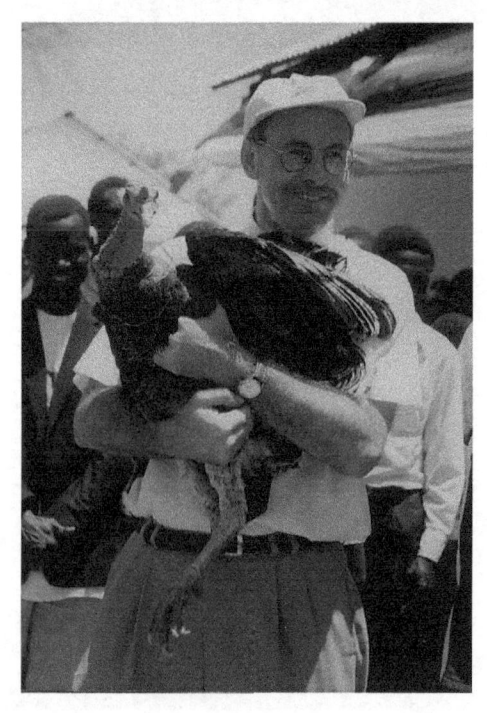

The man from DFID with his turkey

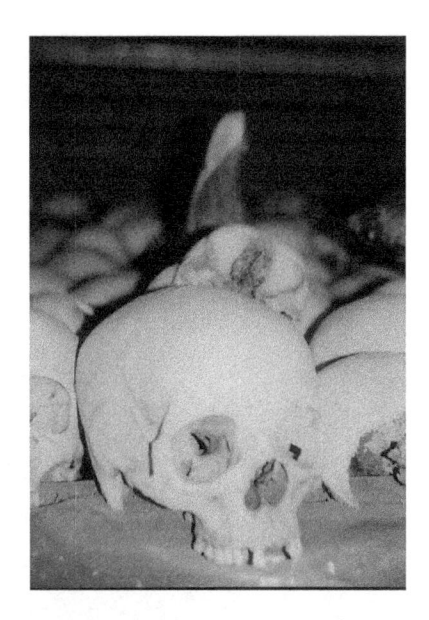

A genocide site in Rwanda

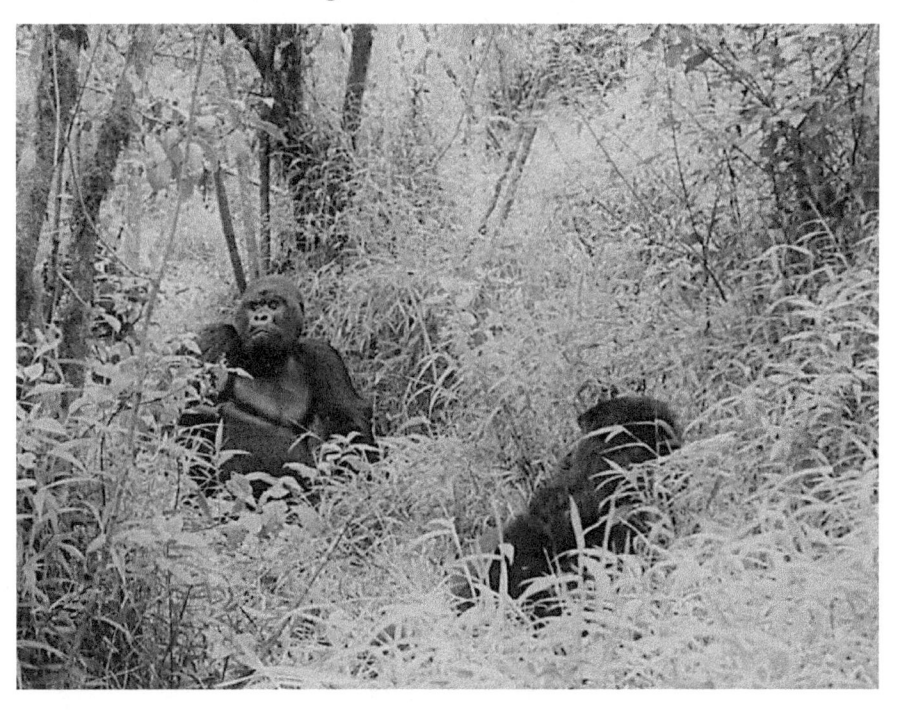

Gorillas in Rwanda

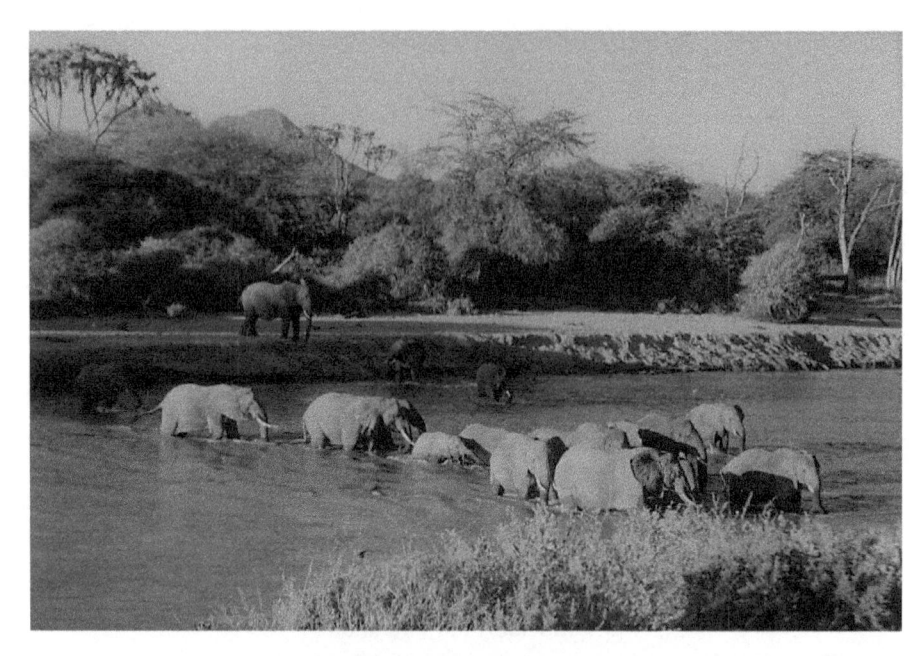

Weekend break in Kenya

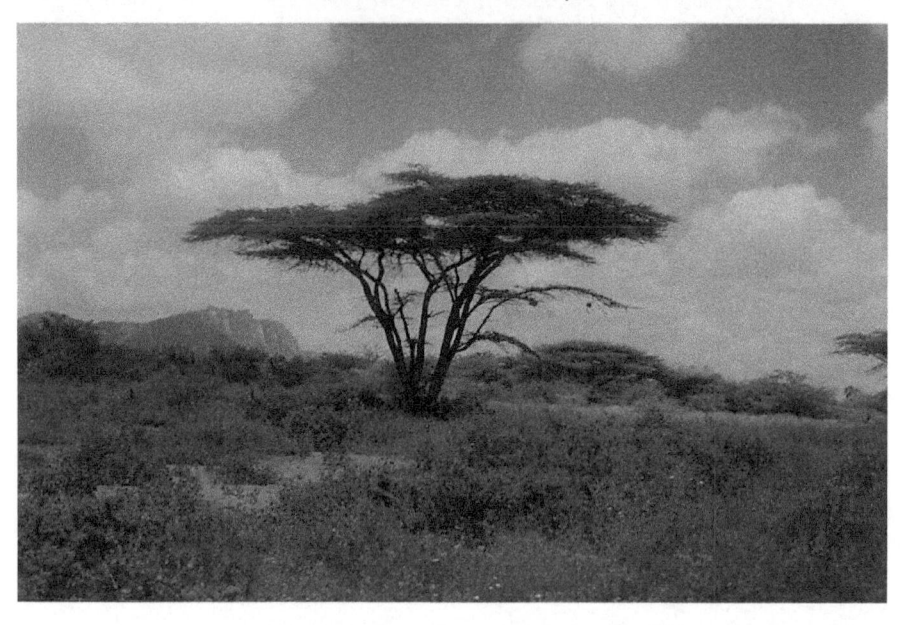

Beautiful Kenya

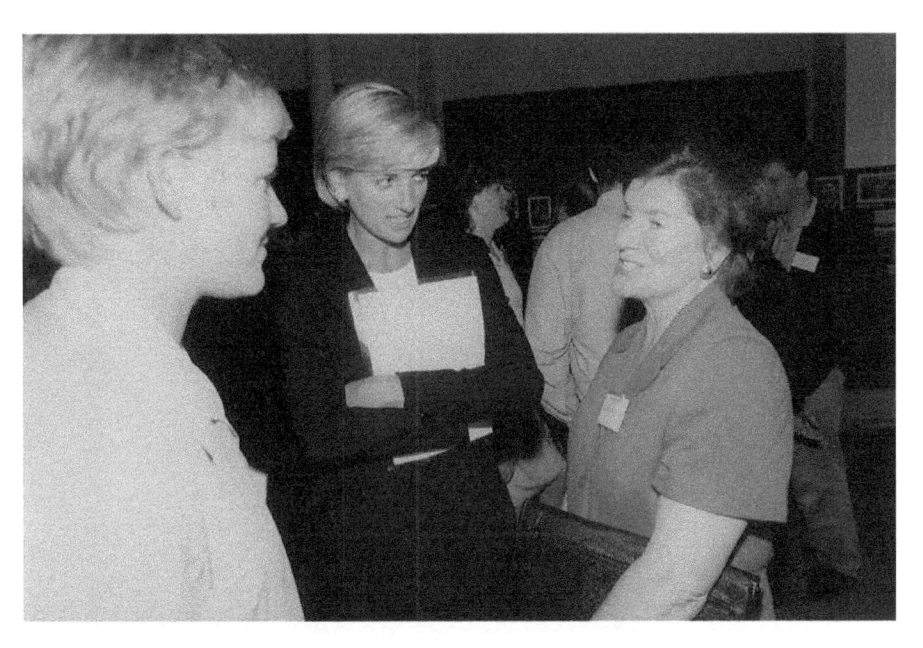

Meeting Princess Diana at The Royal Geographical Society

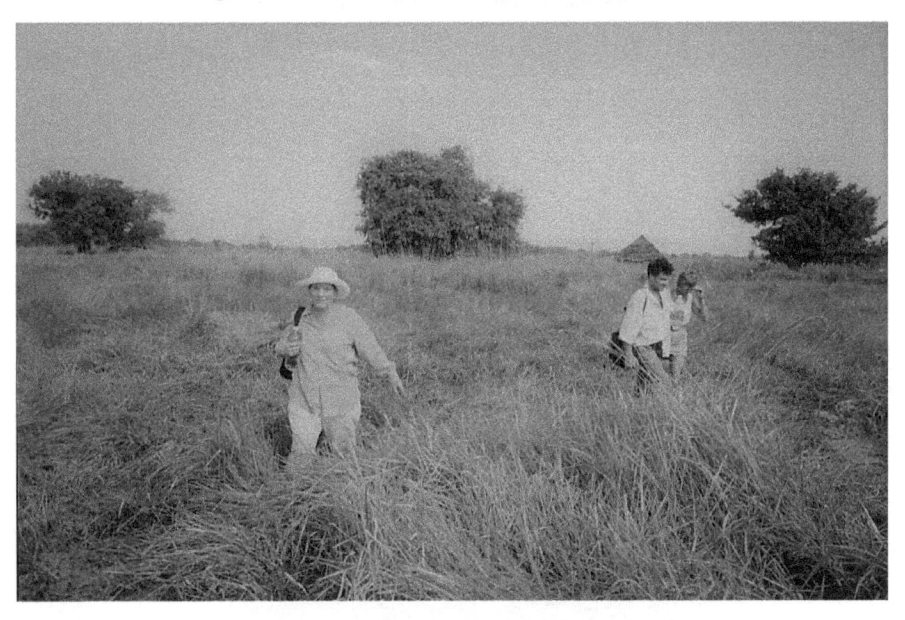

Walking the swamps, South Sudan

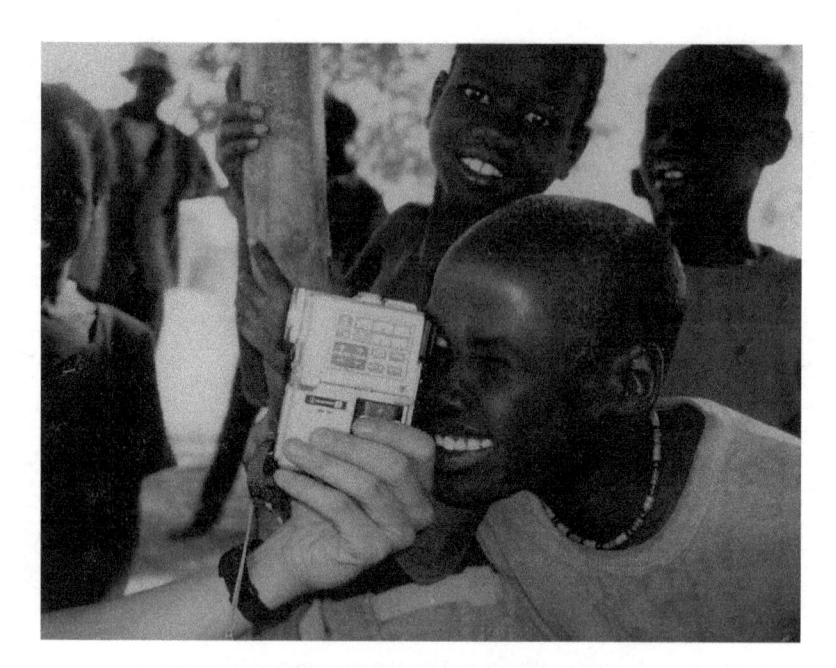

Children in South Sudan inspecting our camera

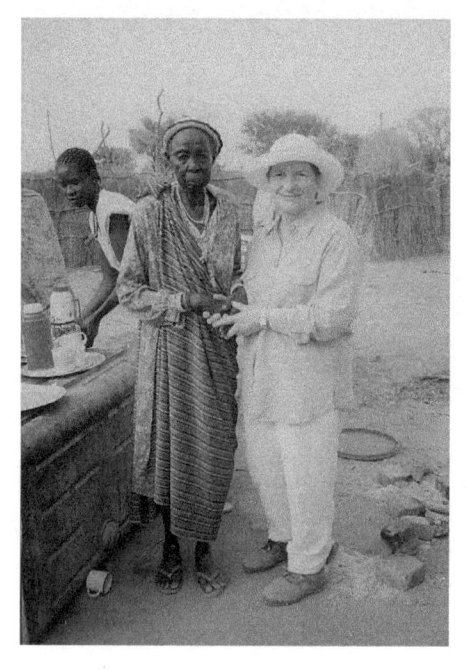

Justin Yak's mother in South Sudan

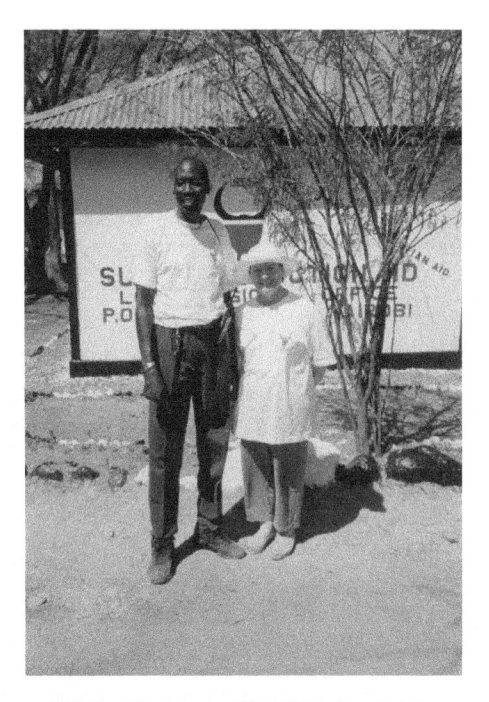

With Achul, my 7ft tall Dinka Guide

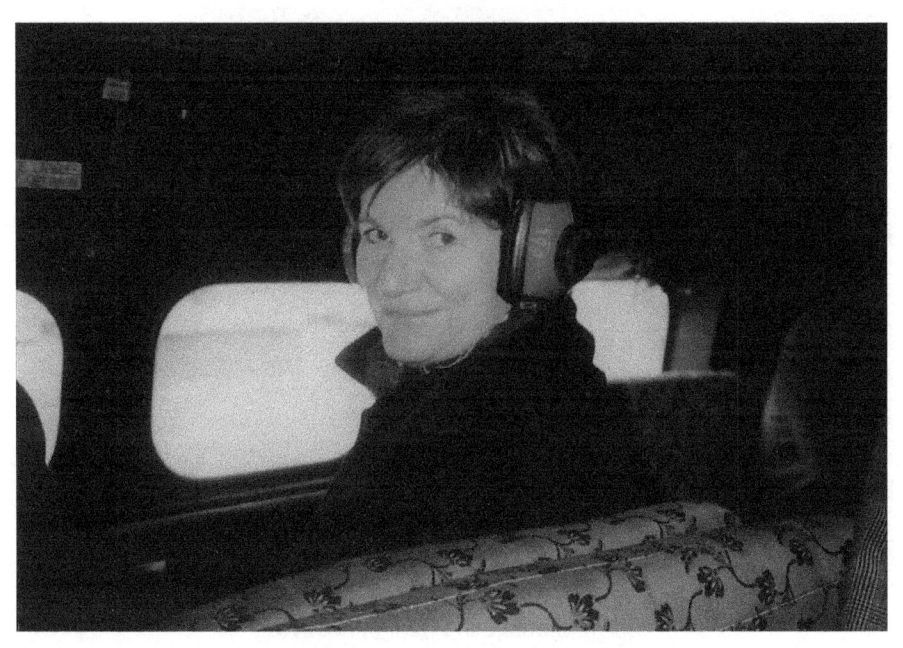

Helicopter ride into Azad Kashmir

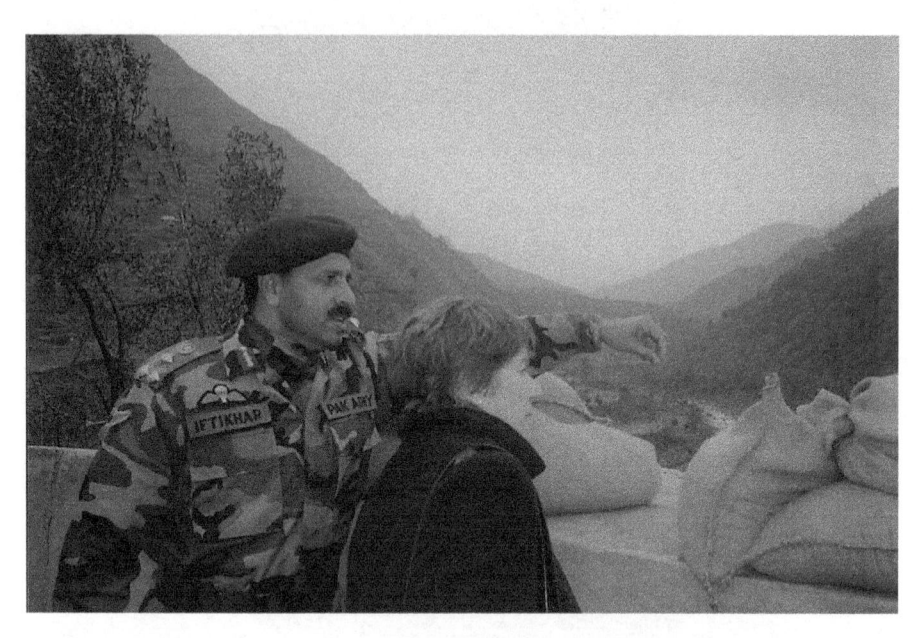

Border trenches between Azad Kashmir and Jammu Kashmir

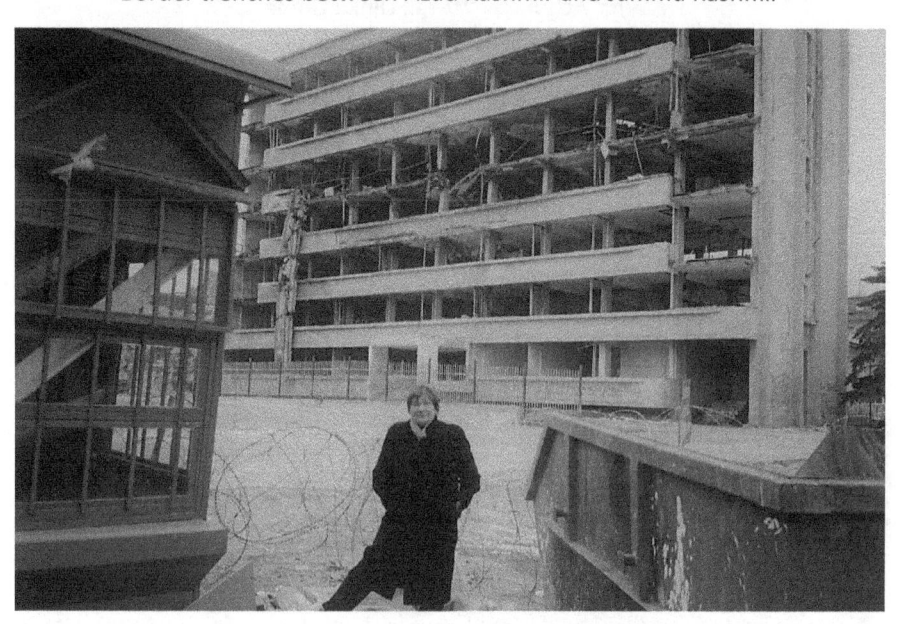

Bomb damage in Pristina, Kosovo

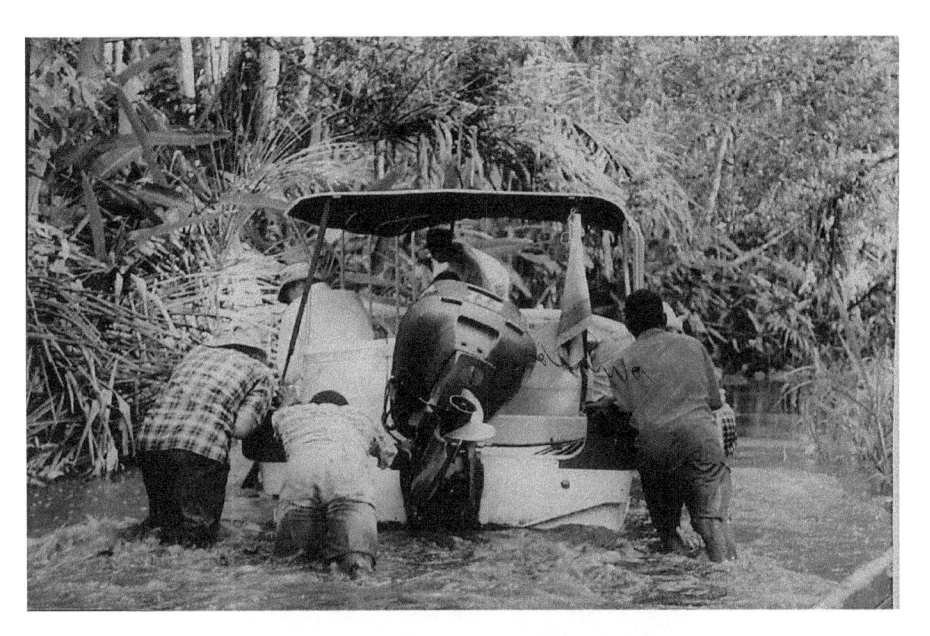

Up river in Colombia

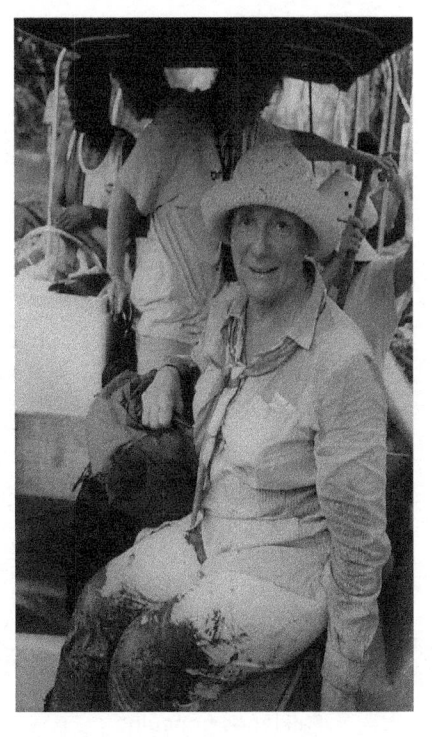

Rescued from the mud in Colombia

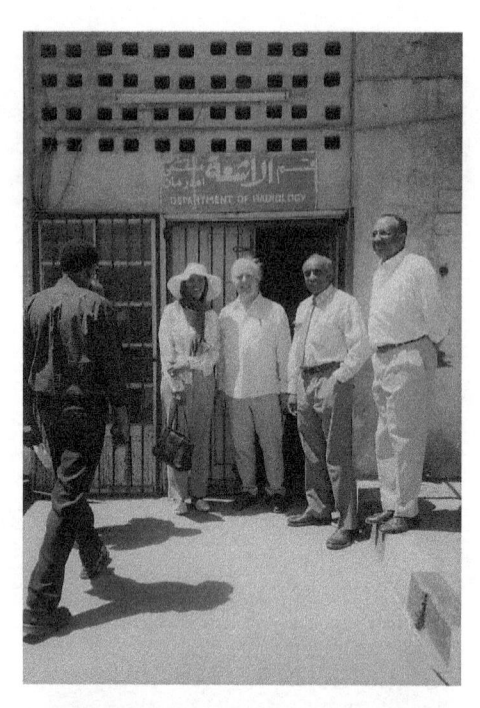

Keith Tonge at the Radiology Department, Omdurman Hospital, Sudan

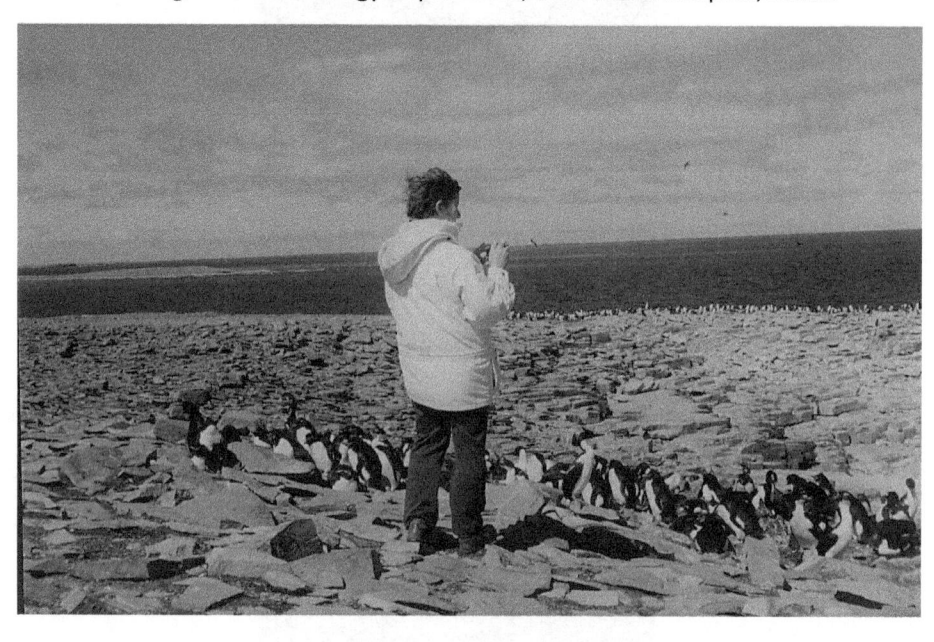

Falklands penguins

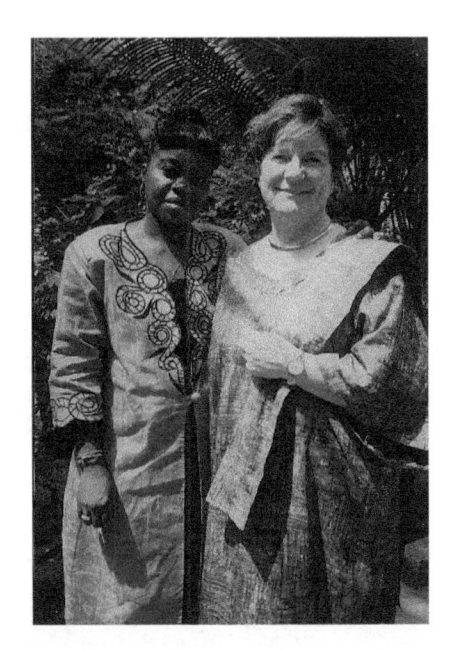

With Satta Amara in Sierra Leone

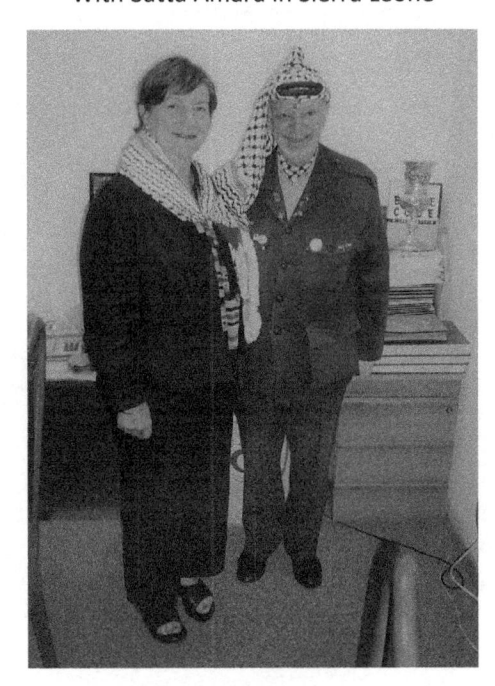

Meeting Yasser Arafat (Photo: Christian Aid)

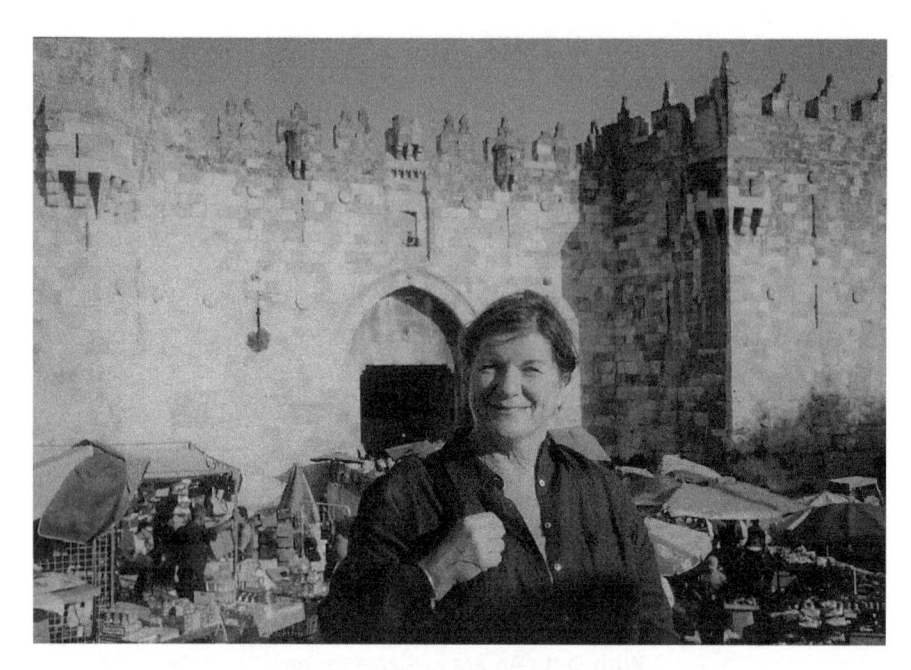

Damascus Gate, Jerusalem (Photo: Christian Aid)

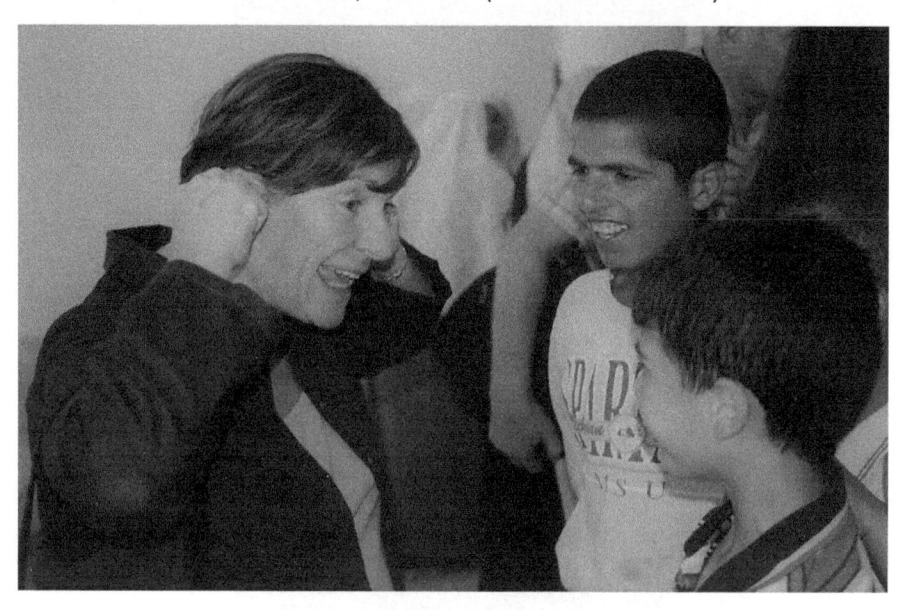

Having fun in Gaza (Photo: Christian Aid)

Chapter 14: The Jewel in the Crown

The Select Committee decided that the study for 1999 would be the position and empowerment of women in developing countries, and India and Bangladesh were chosen to look at this issue. I have never thought of India as 'developing', but it does have the greatest number of the poorest people in the world, despite its apparent success in so many fields, and our Department for International Development was still (at that time) giving much development aid to those people.

Women in India have a lot of influence within their own families, especially in the higher echelons of Indian society. They had a woman Prime Minister long before we did, but everything seemed still to be dictated by caste. The people at the bottom of the pile, the outcasts or Dalits, still struggling to survive, form 15 per cent of the population. Early marriage and dowries seemed to be the main problem for women in India. Education was still taking second place for the girls in most families and like women in many other countries, once married, they become breeding machines until they die. We visited a complex from which girl sex workers operated, often the daughters and granddaughters of women who had earned their living the same way. There we saw efforts by aid agencies to help them achieve a better life. One girl pleaded with me to take her home with me for a better life. Oh, if only I could have done, but all the women there needed a better life. We inspected newly renovated slums, whose residents had been given a clean water supply and neat little rooms to live in. We also met members of the Hijra community, transgender and intersex people who have a special status in India and are accepted by Indian society. Everywhere we went, we were trailed by little boys and beggars, calling us women 'Aunty' and asking for money. Give in, and a mob appears from nowhere demanding the same. When I came home, I read Rohinton Mistry's great novel *A Fine Balance*, which explains it all.

Out of the whole Select Committee membership, only Tony Worthington and I got up before dawn one morning to drive to the Taj Mahal. It seemed crazy to be in India and not allow ourselves that one treat. I suppose, to the well-travelled retired English, the Taj Mahal is just one of those places. It is very special and stunningly beautiful and was worth the early start. Nevertheless, I found what we saw of India to be irritating and frustrating. We were subjected to tirades of 'good news' from officials we met and a huge disdain for us English, especially when one member of the committee criticised the use of child labour. This precipitated an outburst from one minister, telling us that nobody had come along to Great Britain when we were pushing boys up chimneys and making little children pull trucks down mines and ruin their health in unsafe factories. Nobody, he said, interfered with you, so you have no right to criticise us. Phew. Quite right, but it did not help me have any firm impression of what was going on in Indian society. All seemed cloaked in mystery. On our way out from that meeting, the rather old lift in the government building got stuck halfway, and we spent what seemed ages trying to keep spirits up in sweltering heat until rescued. We wondered if it was our punishment for our colonial sins of the past.

The Committee then moved on to Bangladesh, which managed to convey a different impression. Our trip was intended to look at the position and advancement of women, and whilst India seemed more relaxed about its womenfolk, and they were seen all over the cities and countryside, Bangladesh was very different, and we did not see many women in the cities. When our cars were held up in traffic jams, caused by rickshaws in Bangladesh, not cows as in India, we women MPs were subject to close scrutiny as men pressed their noses against the windows of our car and just stared and stared. It was a bit unnerving until we got used to it. Do you smile and acknowledge people in that situation or just stare back? We were told not to respond, so I think we just stared resolutely ahead!

There were signs, however, that Bangladesh was moving in terms of women's rights. All over the country, there were maternal health clinics providing family planning and, although abortion was illegal in Bangladesh, a treatment of 'menstrual regulation' used gentle vacuum aspiration to clear the contents of the uterus when a woman's period was just a few days late. This is legal in Bangladesh and has been since the war of independence from Pakistan in 1971, when rape, as usual, became part of the conflict. This is a procedure that should always have been practised more widely, although it is now being replaced by very effective methods of medical abortion, which do not require hospitalisation at all. The social services NGO, called BRAC (Bangladesh Rehabilitation Assistance Committee), is a semi-official body that delivers all sorts of social care, and my friends at Marie Stopes International were prominent in delivering family planning. I like to think that this emphasis on women's health was due to the two leaders of the rival political parties in Bangladesh, both being women. Sheikh Hasina of the Awami League and Khaleda Zia of the BNP (Bangladesh Nationalist Party) are lifelong bitter enemies, but nevertheless, Bangladesh has done much for its women. The fertility rate there, which used to be around 9 children per family, has now plummeted to 2.1, which means that women and their children can access education. Sheikh Hasina's father, Sheikh Rahman, when he was Prime Minister, was the first to introduce family planning services to Bangladesh about 20 years ago. Sadly he was assassinated by the opposition and is now revered as a national hero. Women are also going to work outside the home in the cities, which is improving the family income and GNP of Bangladesh. These changes are much needed because the country is still hugely overpopulated. When we visited, however, these changes were only just beginning. Outside the cities, women spent their days hidden away in tiny family huts, cooking on fires using dried cow dung as fuel which gave them terrible lung problems, ill health and early death.

Two things, in particular, stand out from that visit unrelated to women's health. Bangladesh stands on the delta of the great river Ganges, which means regular flooding. As global warming progresses and the ice melts in the Himalayas, Bangladesh will gradually sink into the waters of that river. Out in the countryside, we saw a project promoted by DFID called 'meal in a field'. This consisted of a strip of land the size of a small allotment here in England. It was flooded with water, and rice was grown in tidy rows. Between the rows, ducks were paddling and feeding happily, and at the end of each strip was an arched bamboo structure up which peas, beans and any vegetable which would cling grew. The shade provided a cool place for the ducks. On my return, I tried to persuade Keith to try it in his allotment, but foxes were the excuse for not doing so!

That evening, being a long drive from Dhaka, the committee clerks had booked us into the only hotel in the area. It was called the Safeway Motel. That place was a revelation. All the rooms had grand-sounding titles which did not reflect their actual state. Mine was the 'Duchess Suite'. I staggered upstairs and along an unlit corridor to find a room with a large bed covered with filthy, stained nylon sheets, which were a bit of shock in such a humid place. Nevertheless, I thought I would grin, bear it and have a brief rest before we had dinner. I switched on the fan above the bed, which emitted a blue flash before dying altogether. The enormous TV, the only other furniture in the room, did the same thing when I switched it on. Deciding against a rest, I opted for a shower in the alcove attached to the room and made the mistake of going to the loo first and watched sewage come up into the shower tray as I flushed the lavatory. The shower did, however, deliver enough water to wash it down again and cool me off. I recalled how my constituents would call this an MPs' 'jolly'. Grrr.

In the dining room, we were told that they had no cook but that they would send out for a local Chinese takeaway. There was no Bangladeshi food available, sadly and my lemon chicken and rice when it came was definitely not chicken. As I pulled the flesh away from the tiny bones and revealed a delicate ribcage, I decided, with my zoology dissection days in mind, that it was a rodent of some sort. It was food, and it was cooked, so it got eaten. You do not fuss in places where food is scarce, even for visitors. The TV crew who were with us on that trip had shared the experience, and once it was over and we were heading back to Dhaka, laughter reigned as we tried to recall our experiences on camera.

Other trips followed for me to Bangladesh, looking at the plight of the Bihari people who had been left behind after the war which split Bangladesh and Pakistan. They had no civil rights at all and were living in appalling conditions, ignored and reviled by Bangladeshis because they saw them as the enemy. Eventually, they were granted rights and became Bangladeshi citizens, but a hardcore of elderly people remained who had always wanted to go to Pakistan but were rejected by that country.

I saw in very dramatic terms another agony imposed on the people of the sub-continent of India when we left. A Kashmiri-born LibDem activist had been trying to persuade Patsy Calton, LibDem MP for Cheadle in Greater Manchester, to visit Azad Kashmir – the Pakistan-controlled part of Kashmir – and she agreed, provided I came with her. She was not well whilst we were there, and the brief visit during the parliamentary recess, which we paid for ourselves, was very tough. Pakistan and India were still slogging it out as they had done ever since the British led by Lord Mountbatten had left the problem behind. A plebiscite for self-determination of this Muslim majority had been promised but never happened. We saw trenches and sandbags reminiscent of the First World War dug along the border, with Indian trenches across no man's land 50 yards away, on the Jammu Kashmir border. Soldiers were pointing guns at each other in time-honoured fashion. When will they ever learn?

We managed to record the poverty out in the countryside, and the glorious luxury of the old governors' residence in Lahore with its silk-lined walls, before we left. Thankfully the residence is now within the grounds of a girls' higher education college. Patsy was ill, and I was glad to get her back home. She was a heroic woman and a fine MP, diagnosed with a vicious form of breast cancer shortly afterwards. At her team's request, she campaigned in a wheelchair all through the 2005 general election, increasing her majority by a considerable margin, but sadly died soon afterwards.

Chapter 15: Off the SCID

After the trip to India and Pakistan, the party leaders decided that it was a bit of a heavy schedule for me to be party spokesman for International Development and be a member of the Select Committee for International Development (SCID), and I suspect one of the boys wanted a turn, so I was replaced. I was very sad to leave, but it did relieve the pressure somewhat and allowed me to spend more time with my constituents, which I have to say were being very well served by my office staff in Richmond. Nick Carthew and Serena Hennessy, both of whom were and had been local councillors, dealt with the relentless casework which pours into all MPs' offices, and the late Polly Wright, who acted as my diary secretary, made sure I did not miss any local events. There is always that occasion though when attending a local orchestra concert or a school play when somebody says how good it is to see you 'relaxing'. The family gets neglected. I did not see enough of my new grandson, and other babies were coming to give us a total of seven lovely grandchildren by 2010.

In the New Year, I was to go with Harriet Harman and Teresa Gorman to look at sex and relationship education in the Netherlands. A large number of women MPs in parliament were very interested in this issue and keen to bring in proper education in this field for all schools in the UK. At that time, we had the highest teenage pregnancy rate in Europe, and the Netherlands had the lowest. Labour's Harriet Harman had been the first woman to bring her babies into Westminster, and I think, was famous once for feeding one of them in a committee room. Why on earth not? Feeding a baby does not require great academic skills, after all. Being an MP does not either come to think of it. Teresa Gorman was a Tory supporter of women's rights and reproductive rights in particular. I remember her once telling me that nothing would make her stop taking HRT, which we both agreed had transformed the pesky menopause for many women, even though some doctors, male ones, in particular, liked to discourage its use. Must keep the women under control, of course. Teresa's husband had told her he would put what was left of her HRT prescription into her coffin with her if she died first, in case she needed it in the afterlife.

We sat in on some wonderful sex education lessons and watched a totally unembarrassed and cheerful teacher show the mixed group of boys and girls how to use a condom – using a model, of course! She then distributed condoms to every pupil and told them that their 'homework' was to learn how they were used. It was no good, she said, trying to use a condom when they had sex for the first time. They must practise first. All attendees at sexual health (family planning) clinics in the Netherlands are encouraged to go 'double-dutch', meaning using a method like the pill to prevent pregnancy and condoms to prevent infection. We were encouraging this in our clinics in the UK too, but we were thwarted time and time again in our efforts to make sex education compulsory in our schools.

Governments never want to offend religious groups, and so it was left to the school governors to decide. It was 2018 before we got this measure through both houses of parliament. Two years on, and the government is still consulting with schools. We are nearly there. Twenty years trying to curb teenage pregnancies and young people being abused sexually because they did not have the confidence or knowledge to resist. Religion has a lot to answer for.

Women's health featured again when I was asked to go with a small charity to Albania to look at the condition of children there. It was during the bombing of Serbia and the fleeing of people from Kosovo who were being attacked by the Serbs coming south. Kosovans are Muslim, Serbs are on the whole Christian, although at this time they were not practising it – behaviour not exclusive to Serbs I may say.

In Albania, I was asked to visit the hospital where many violated women and their children had ended up. I learned under the greatest secrecy of the terrible rapes these women had suffered, often with broken bottles or rifle butts, injuries they could not tell their families about for fear of rejection. Raped by so-called Christians and rejected by so-called Muslims. We did what we could. After seeing and hearing what I had so far in Rwanda, Sudan and now the Balkans, it became increasingly clear to me that rape was part of ethnic cleansing and genocide, although this was not generally accepted by the international bodies at that time. More cheering were the visits to ordinary homes in Tirana, where there was a family in every room, not necessarily related to the people living in the house. 'They are our brothers and sisters,' we were told. 'We must help them.' Have our people been as welcoming to people fleeing war and persecution in recent years?

Later in the year, I was back in the region with the Inter-Parliamentary Union, one week after the end of the Kosovo War, and experienced the chaos of post-war Pristina. Cheering people in the streets, car horns blaring and graffiti on walls proclaiming, 'Thank you, Bill Clinton. Thank you, Tony Blair.' Even, 'Thank you, Robin Cook.' Was it this adulation that gave Blair the sense that whatever he did was good and righteous and led to disastrous events in Afghanistan and Iraq in particular?

Pristina was cheerful but packed out with stolen cars driven by anyone who could lay hands on one. The Serbs had ripped number plates off cars so that nobody could claim ownership. It was a free for all and a mighty traffic jam. After several meetings with potential members of the parliament of the new Kosovo, we tried and failed to get back to the airstrip for our RAF flight home. We were royally entertained by a rather delicious army captain with beautiful green eyes, who plied us with whisky and his wife's shortbread whilst he summoned a helicopter from Skopje to take us there for a 'commercial' flight home. Skopje airport was seething with refugees, but the following day we squeezed onto a smoke-filled plane bound for Zurich. Unfortunately, this was held up because the pilot would not go until he had filled the plane! As a consequence, we missed the planned connection to Heathrow and had to negotiate and wait yet again for a flight to Paris then home. Luggage arrived torn and battered a few days later, but I was home.

It had taken around 36 hours.

Throughout this year, the main issue in my constituency, as ever, had been the threat of yet another terminal at Heathrow Airport. Aircraft noise makes south-west London very miserable indeed. Heathrow developed by accident in the post-war years, and BAA was always seeking to expand capacity on the grounds that it was good for London and the economy. A group had been set up to fight the expansion, and I was president for some years. We battled Terminal 4 to no avail, and this was soon followed by a fight to stop Terminal 5, even though we had been promised after T4 that there would be no more expansion. As everyone now knows, T5 was built, and after more promises and before the ink was dry on the documents, an application was made for a third runway at Heathrow. This is now in its final stages before implementation, and one wonders just where this will stop. To have the biggest airport in the world in an area where flights taking off and landing cross the most heavily populated part of the UK just seems madness. Madness was the word also used to describe Boris Johnson's scheme to build a new airport in the Thames estuary, but it always seemed to me to be the sanest suggestion that man ever made.

Nevertheless, in November of my first year off the Select Committee, I was in a party, flying, yes flying, to the Falklands Islands via Ascension Island in a rickety RAF transport plane. Our brief was to see what many of our soldiers and sailors had died to defend in Mrs Thatcher's publicity stunt against Galtieri, who was President of Argentina at the time. My teenage son and his friends were so fired up over this that they slept outside the Albert Hall that September before the Last Night of the Proms and managed to persuade a doorman to let them in to indulge in a bit of loud singing and patriotism. I was not told until the next day.

The trip was funded by the government of this tiny dependent territory. It is a group of flat, windswept moorland islands, peppered with sheep and wonderful wildlife, but very few people indeed, around three thousand when we were there. They appeared to live life in the same way as I did as a child in the 1950s. Old fashioned and stubbornly British, but defended by a hugely expensive garrison paid for by us. After 16, their children were educated back in England, in a sixth form college in Winchester, and it just seemed such an odd situation. We spent millions defending this for what? At the time, most of us in the group thought it was taking national pride a bit far and that the islands, being so close to Argentina, could rightly be theirs and called 'Las Malvinas'. There were whisperings of oil exploration, but the members of the government there were dismissive of this and were concentrating on fisheries which were and still are the main income of the islands. Of course, the whisperings were right and had probably reached Mrs Thatcher's ears at the time of the Falklands War. There are oil reserves there worth exploiting, though they are proving difficult and expensive for the companies involved. How many lives have been lost in the last two hundred years in our thirst for oil?

On Christmas Day 1999, we were all having fun when my senior daughter-in-law expressed her concerns about her sister, who was ill with flu over in Kingston. She did not want to go to see her because she was about five months pregnant and naturally worried that she might catch the flu, which was doing the rounds. I volunteered to go and found Linda, a dear girl and a social worker, semi-conscious and blue. She was very ill, indeed.

I called the ambulance and went with her to Kingston Hospital Casualty Department, which was overcrowded and infested (I use that word advisedly) with drunks and minor injuries, which as a former Casualty Officer, makes me very angry indeed. Despite the best efforts of the team, who eventually came to Linda through the chaos and transferred her to Intensive Care, she died in the early hours of Boxing Day, surrounded by her family, who had been summoned. The flu virus had attacked her heart muscle, and her young heart stopped forever. She was in her early thirties. All thoughts of politics and Christmas melted away. Two families devastated by the death of a wonderful young woman. Millennium Eve, which we had all been eagerly awaiting, just seemed so pointless. Fireworks, signifying nothing except that familiar long haul through bereavement and back to normality without a family member. If any good came out of that death, it was that Ed Davey, the LibDem MP for Kingston, and I renewed our efforts to get a new Casualty Department at Kingston, which had been sorely needed for years.

We were fortunate to have Frank Dobson as Secretary of State for Health, who cared, and a Labour government determined to invest in hospitals and new schools, which they did. Yes, I know there was criticism of the way they were funded with PFI, but we got them, and we should never forget the good that was done by that government, despite its mistakes on foreign policy later on. They transformed our health and social services and schools. Kingston Hospital got its new Casualty Department. It should have been called the Linda Wing. Neither was it this expenditure that caused the national deficit, which Tories like to bang on about! That deficit was caused by the money we had to borrow to bail out the banks after years of 'light touch management' introduced by the Thatcher government. Apologies for that short rant.

In the new year, I was invited to Namibia to a women's parliamentarians' conference. At the time, they had more women in their parliament than we did, a sore point for many of us. It was a smart, clean country. Something to do with the German colonisation? I don't know, but there was a sense of order there despite the terrible poverty you find all over Africa. I ate bush meat with a man from DFID – just to say I had – and I had been given the lovely task of taking his grandmother's engagement ring out to David Blomfield's son Rupert who had become engaged while working out there on a VSO project.

The year 2000 was most memorable, however, for a quite terrifying visit to Colombia. My researcher at the time was a brilliant Kew girl called Alice Hutchinson. She appeared to work in a sort of zany chaos all around her, laughing along as she did so. She was nevertheless the most efficient researcher and persuasive too because although I was trying to resist more trips abroad than I needed, she got me interested in the scandal of the drugs trade worldwide and the scourge those drugs were to developing countries. So it was that I found myself on my way to Colombia, courtesy of a voluntary organisation called Peace Brigades International, with two other MPs and a young envoy sent by the Archbishop of Canterbury. It did not really help that, following a reading of Louis de Bernières' *Captain Corelli's Mandolin*, I had followed up with his Latin American trilogy, which includes *The Troublesome Offspring of Cardinal Guzman*, which is a fairly gory and scary book about the drugs trade in South America. It did not help either that as we left Heathrow, I was developing a humdinger of a head cold with a fever too, so I was in an impressionable state.

As I ran through all my boxes and colleagues' boxes of tissues, we sat through meetings about the failure of the rule of law in Colombia and the problems caused by the left-wing and brutal rebels called the FARC and the equally brutal and troublesome group called the ELN. Both groups destroyed villages in the countryside if the people did not do as they wished, which was to grow coca for the drugs trade and to fund their arms purchases. The violence had spread into the cities. The next day we were to fly to Medellín, which was the stronghold of the chief of all the rebels, the legendary Pablo Escobar. He was so wealthy from the coca trade that he had built a metro system on stilts all around his city, and Medellín had consequently been referred to as 'The Silver Bowl'. It was certainly that as our plane flew over-preparing to land – a stunningly beautiful sight in the moonlight. We were packed off to our rooms and told to stay there until fetched by our guides in the morning, and I slumped into bed wondering why the TV seemed to be on somewhere because there was the constant noise of shouting and gunfire. I soon realised that this was Medellín at night! The gunfire was all outside in the streets of the city. I must have snatched a few hours of sleep, and thankfully I had stopped streaming from the nose.

After more meetings the next day, we were transferred to Turbo, which is around 340 kilometres from Medellín and was regarded then as the hub of the cocaine trade. It is a small port offering transfers across the Gulf of Uraba for backpackers wishing to go on to Panama. Certainly, none of them wanted to go where we were going. We crossed the water to the mouth of the Atrato River leading into the jungle, where we were to visit a tiny community that had relocated themselves to be self-sufficient with the help of Peace Brigades International. The agreement with the Ejército de Liberación Nacional (ELN, or National Liberation Army of Columbia), in this case, was to leave them in peace to keep chickens and practice subsistence farming. They would not have to grow coca, and they would not have any arms.

To get there, we had to take a boat up the river through the jungle. Unfortunately, after an hour or so, the river was getting too shallow for the boat – this, they explained, was due to illegal logging in that area, which was causing the river to silt up. Eventually, it was suggested we get out of the boat and plough through the jungle in our welly boots as the two boatmen punted the boat through the mud until we could get back on board. I had never realised how noisy jungles are. Every sort of creature was saying something; monkeys were chattering and swinging about, birds screeching, and the incessant hum and buzz of insects. After half an hour or so, we came to a dead halt because our way was completely blocked by a hornet's nest, which even us Londoners knew should not be disturbed. We were told to walk to the river, and the boat would try to pick us up for a short stretch, but on the way, I sank into mud which quickly started to suck me down. I was bodily lifted out of it by a Tory saviour, Gary Streeter, leaving one welly behind to be consumed by the mud monster.

We progressed in this way for hours until we reached the 'village', which was a collection of rough awnings and small huts around a long wooden structure raised from the ground, which was the sleeping quarters for the whole village. We hosed down, some swam in the river that had nearly defeated us, and we were given fried eggs and rough bread, which was one of the most delicious meals I had ever tasted. Before bed, we listened to stories of the lives of the villagers. A horrific incident had taken place a week before when the ELN had come in and accused the headman of some misdemeanour or other, and his head had been cut off, and the children were forced to play a ghoulish game of football with it, watched by their tormentors. I realised that the ghastly imagery in *The Troublesome Offspring of Cardinal Guzman* was not all from the imagination of Louis de Bernières.

On a public health note – my medical training never deserts me – the dugout latrine and the stockade around it was squeaky clean, smothered in quicklime inside and outside the pit so that no insects invaded. Wonderful! We slept that night in wooden cots vacated for us by some of the villagers, in the long hut with everyone else. In a cot next to me, there was a mother and two tiny, malnourished children. On the other side was a very amorous couple, not at all deterred from their activities by members of parliament from the UK enjoying their performance. Dogs roamed round our beds and came in and out of the hut and occasionally barked during the night. I don't remember lying awake for long. It had been a hard day. The next morning another, flatter boat materialised to take us back to the river mouth, not before a stop on the way to look at the activities of loggers destroying the forest. We were not convinced that the experiment of safe villages was working!

The travails of Jenny Tonge were not quite over. We were transported back to Turbo across the sea in a speed boat, and I and a fellow woman MP were put in the back. The driver went so fast that the back of the boat was half underwater most of the way, and we arrived completely drenched. Better than the river, though, and it was so hot we soon dried off. The final thrill for us was our overnight accommodation in Turbo. I was put in a room on the ground floor near reception. There was a bed, a chest of drawers and a shower in one corner surrounded by an old plastic curtain.

Never mind if the door didn't lock, I was near reception.

In the middle of the night, there was crashing, shouting and the usual gunfire. I pushed the chest of drawers against my door and stood in the shower with the curtain drawn until it was quiet – just in case! Apparently, the receptionist was on some gang's wanted list and had been 'taken out' during the night. It was good to be returning to Bogota that day and then home. When I got back to Kew, I was the butt of lots of jokes from my husband. I was smothered in assorted insect bites, and unaccountably, I developed a shedding scalp for weeks afterwards, the joys of a short stay in the South American rain forests.

Whatever else that trip did, it convinced me that the way we deal with drugs is wrong, but the demand continues, and the trade across the world causes untold suffering for people who have no other option but to obey the drug lords and grow the stuff. It's the drug lords and the middlemen who flourish while we criminalise young 'mules' and addicts. The same no doubt applies to heroin cultivation in Afghanistan. If the smart snorters of cocaine in the City and others could spend a few days seeing what we saw on that trip, they would think again.

Much more happened in this year 2000 but nothing more important than the birth of two more grandchildren. Our family was growing!

Chapter 16: Big Smoke 9/11

There was one huge event in 2001 that changed the world. Before it occurred, however, there were the usual adventures in the constituency and abroad. Heathrow, and the fact that my constituency lies under its flight path, was highlighted when the Chair of the Kew Society, Malcolm Welchman, was hit by a lump of ice whilst he was walking down Kew Road. It was identified as coming from the contents of a toilet compartment being jettisoned before landing a plane. It was doubly insulting because Malcolm and his wife Julia had been doughty campaigners against the expansion of Heathrow Airport for years. Julia was a schoolteacher and quite rightly concerned about the effect of the continual noise overhead. It was not an isolated incident, and work started to identify the airline.

Over the same few months, two bodies fell from the sky, one through the roof of a local school, luckily injuring no one, and another in the car park of our local Sainsbury's. These events were harder to deal with because the bodies were desperate people trying to escape poverty and persecution in some faraway land and deciding to take the risk of stowing away in the undercarriages of planes whilst they were on the runway. It is difficult to imagine how desperate someone must be to do that. Did they really think they had a chance of survival?

Another battle was being fought over graffiti which were appearing all over the area, grossly offending the sensibilities of the people of Richmond and Kingston. A local artist had voluntarily painted murals on both sides of the pedestrian bridge over the railway at Kew, which stopped graffiti appearing there, but a few years later, Network Rail declared that these rather nice pictures were not in keeping with their 'image' whatever that was and had it painted over so that the graffiti artists had a clean slate. By that time, the youth of the area were moving on to other pastimes, on their computers, no doubt. I spent an afternoon in the Lords listening to a debate on the Morning After Pill being available over the counter, which was being challenged by noble Lords who thought they should maintain control of the bodies of the nation's women. It was defeated, and to this day, women can obtain this remedy if they pay at a pharmacy or free from their GP.

I had to make another quick visit to Sudan at the time of the Queen Mother's death, so I never saw the pomp of that occasion, though Keith did. He was persuaded by his secretary at St Thomas' Hospital to give her a quick tour in the Commons in their lunch hour: they reached Westminster Hall as the last household guard was taking up his position at the corner of the coffin after the candles had been lit. They were the first people to witness this Royal lying in state. It made me quite popular amongst Keith's staff.

As I was flying out of Heathrow, a minor storm was breaking because, some hours before, I had told a radio programme that I believed certain drugs should be legalised, and the purified products sold at registered outlets in the same way that alcohol is. The newspapers loved it. Madwoman doctor MP who had seen enough drug addicts in her time as a casualty officer to last a lifetime, actually daring to suggest that less damage would be done to individuals and society, let alone people in the drug-growing areas of the world, if the drug trade was brought under control. The arguments raged. I was ticked off but did not repent. I have the same opinion today and so do many others, but politicians are terrified of the media and one newspaper – the Daily Mail – in particular.

One picture memory of that trip to Sudan stays in my mind. One afternoon we came back to the little community centre set up by one of the NGOs and saw a crowd of Sudanese men gathered around a flickering TV in the corner, powered by the NGO's own generator. Poverty-stricken people, standing in their dusty white robes, watched the Queen Mother's funeral in complete amazement. I would have loved to have talked at length to them afterwards, but we were heading off out again. What on earth did they make of it? The older ones, no doubt with reverence. We were often told by Sudanese that things were much better when the British were in control and wanted us back. Others must have looked on in disgust. That night I slept or tried to sleep in a traditional cone-shaped hut on a raised truckle bed under my own mosquito net. As I was dropping off to sleep, I heard a scuffling sound, switched on my torch, and watched a mouse being chased by a scorpion, tail held aloft, across the dirt floor of the hut. I fell asleep!

On my return, we got stuck into the General Election campaign, which had been delayed because of foot-and-mouth disease. Tony Blair's Labour won again, and we made a few more gains under the leadership of Charles Kennedy, whose campaign chair was Tim Razzall, a colleague from Richmond Council days. Tim masterminded the campaign brilliantly and managed a difficult to manage party leader in Charles Kennedy, who was battling demons even then.

Constituency events crowded out the calendar, with a brief duty trip back to Kenya to talk about successful methods of local campaigning. I am never sure that LibDem methods of campaigning are necessarily appropriate for developing countries, but they always love one story I tell about what we used to refer to as the 'Blue Letters'. These letters were handwritten by candidates about policies etc., and then photocopied and put into blue envelopes with the elector's name and address handwritten by teams of helpers – we had many such. I once met Princess Alexandra, who lives in Richmond Park, at a local function, and she told me how she had loved the blue letter because she seldom got handwritten letters anymore, and she thought it was such a treat! A treat until she realised it was yet another leaflet dressed up as a letter. She thoroughly endorsed them, though, and audiences can be impressed!

The parliamentary year drew to a close, and we all looked forward to a rest. We were having just that in southern France and had been on a picturesque train journey up onto the Massif Central for lunch with friends. On the way back, we wearily piled into the car to take us back to our holiday home and heard on the radio that there had been some sort of plane crash in the USA.

It was the 11th of September, but we did not know then quite what an event it was. We can all remember and can bore for England telling 'where we were' when it happened, as we do for the deaths of John F. Kennedy and Princess Diana, but this really was different. The Americans had been gunning for Osama bin Laden since the American Embassy in Kenya had been bombed in 1998 with over 200 people killed. We had discussed it at the LibDem Foreign Affairs meetings but thought it was the Americans looking for an enemy. After 9/11, we began to take them seriously. Al Qaeda became the enemy, and George Bush went on television to talk about a 'crusade', which was one of the most inflammatory words he could have used. Keith screamed at the radio when he heard him and roared, 'That's it. You *stupid* man. Just the word to inflame the Middle East.' Keith spent several years of his childhood in Iraq with his RAF parents, and he loved and remained fascinated by Iraq and the whole of the Middle East for all of his life. His other love, apart from his family, was growing things, following in the footsteps of his mother's family, who were farmers in Dorset. And sailing. His allotment and his boat kept him happy whilst I was out campaigning.

The LibDem party conference gathered soon afterwards, and we were asked to approve a motion supporting the USA in their plan to bomb Afghanistan, where they had decided Osama bin Laden must be. This heralded my first rebellion against my party and leader and engendered a lot of fury from the previous leader too. As International Development spokesperson, I had been receiving reports from the NGOs in Afghanistan of the famine there and the vulnerability of the people. Bombing would be unthinkable. The supporters argued that it would be 'precision bombing' of the cave fortress where they thought bin Laden was with thousands of men; my colleagues were gung-ho about it. My understanding was that there was a huge network of caves, and they were unlikely to kill bin Laden even if, at this stage, it would help. It was also suggested that the Afghan Taliban government had been given three weeks to hand him over, and they had not complied; therefore, the bombing was ordered.

I did not understand, and still do not understand that, to use a simple analogy, if you want to find a needle (bin Laden) in a haystack (the Tora Bora caves), you do not bomb the haystack. That way, you spread whatever you are bombing over a much wider area. Patience is needed, and as hundreds of thousands of people were starving in Afghanistan, I proclaimed in my speech to the conference that we should be dropping food on Afghanistan, not bombs. The people there were not responsible for 9/11. This brought the sky down on my head because I was just a naive woman and did not understand these things. Nevertheless, some people there who agreed with me went out and got T-shirts printed saying 'Food not bombs' and wore them for the rest of the conference—my first rebellion.

A couple of months later, our fourth grandchild was born to the ever-expanding Tonge family.

Chapter 17: Return to Africa

The gathering storm which was to end in the invasion of Iraq dominated a lot of political debate in 2002, as did the continuing bombardment of Afghanistan. The American President was on a roll, presumably fired by the self-righteousness he shared with Tony Blair, but before any decisions were taken, I was busy on all sorts of fronts – especially Africa. Before my next visit to that continent, I had a minor personal victory and brief celebrity. I have always worried about faith schools and wish that all state education was secular, with parents taking care of the religious education of their children. I recognised, however, that it would be a huge expense to take state control of all the Anglican and Catholic schools in the UK, especially as they were popular with parents. There was a move towards state schools becoming academies and local authorities losing their control over them.

I was incensed one night, listening on the car radio that Creationism was being taught in state schools in the northeast of England, the schools being sponsored by a local businessman. As a scientist and Darwinist, I was appalled, and luckily I had a Prime Minister's question the following day, which I used to ask Tony Blair if he was happy that Creationism was being taught in those state schools. Astonishingly he replied that he was perfectly happy because those schools were providing children with a good education and getting good exam results. His reply, I am glad to say, was not received well, and many columnists took up the topic in the newspapers; as a result, I was immortalised by getting a mention in Richard Dawkins' book, *The God Delusion*. Well, my grandchildren approve of the mention anyway!

During the 2001 General Election, I had been asked by the Commonwealth Parliamentary Association to host a politician from Sierra Leone and allow her to campaign with me and experience our methods of electioneering. Her name was Satta Amara. She had founded and was Secretary-General of '50/50', a campaign to get more women involved in politics in Sierra Leone, which was just coming out of the most terrible civil war which had lasted for nearly ten years. It was finally ended by Blair ordering British troops into Sierra Leone to stop the fighting. It was a successful campaign in much the same way as the action in Kosovo had been and no doubt swelled his ego a little more. The people of Sierra Leone were so grateful he became a hero there. Satta came over to Richmond, and we had great fun campaigning together, although, by our standards, she was incredibly slow.

We would sweep down a road knocking on doors, trying to find out as quickly as possible where our vote lay. One evening I had finished one side of my road and turned round to see that Satta was only on her third call. Her idea of canvassing was to talk at length about politics, women, wars, religion, Sierra Leone – anything but finding out how a person would vote. She was charming, though, and we loved her, and she did pick up a few tricks. She was given a constituency to fight at the next election in Sierra Leone. This was in the dangerous area that contained the diamond fields, the 'blood diamonds' which were the main cause of the civil war. I suppose her party leaders thought a woman was expendable.

Anyway, Satta invited me to Sierra Leone this year to meet and talk to the aspiring women politicians there. I travelled alone, which I have to say was a little daunting. The airport for Freetown was across the sea from the city itself, and I had to wait for a helicopter to take me to where I was being met outside 'customs'.

There was a huge crush on the helicopter, which far exceeded its maximum capacity, and I was a bit concerned as we took off when several men ran across the tarmac, threw bags and cases into the non-existent space (one landed on my lap) and jumped in or hung on for the trip. We flew just above the water, I can only suppose because the machine was so overloaded it could not get higher, but a smiling Satta was there to greet me and explain that that was 'normal' for Sierra Leone. She also presented me with the national dress she had sewn for me for the big meeting the next day. I looked ridiculous and was too hot but needs must. Never criticise the politician who does apparently stupid things when abroad – it is often done so as not to offend the hosts!

My role was to meet the women who were brave enough to have joined Satta's campaign, and I learned once again the difficulties of doing anything when you have endless pregnancies to cope with. Family planning was practically non-existent in Sierra Leone then. How can women gain control in their country when they have no control over their own bodies?

At an afternoon meeting, I met some victims of the civil war who had had limbs amputated by the RUF (Revolutionary United Front) rebel soldiers backed by the infamous President of Liberia, Charles Taylor. The victims were asked whether they wanted 'short or long sleeves', meaning amputation above or below the elbow. I learned about blood diamonds on that trip too and supported the campaign which led to the Kimberley Process, crafted in part by Robin Cook, to ensure that diamonds are properly certificated at source, and illegal diamonds such as blood diamonds could not be sold to fund wars.

Passing through the various check-in desks as I left for the airport on the way home, and officials wrote on bits of paper and scribbled their authority on my bag. I could not resist, as I reached a very cheerful and jovial soldier at the last hurdle, asking him if he was going to ask me if I wanted to buy diamonds? He looked from side to side and motioned me round the back of the shed. I did not go, regretting my own sense of humour, which has always got me into trouble. It was a short stay in what could be such a lovely country, but where over 70 per cent of the population live below the poverty line, and there are virtually no health services. Despite massive UK aid going into Sierra Leone after the war ended, no health systems were in place to stop the spread of the deadly Ebola virus twelve years later. Too much emphasis on hospitals and glamorous services and not enough simple public health networks?

In 2004 my friend Satta Amara died with 23 others in a helicopter crash on her way to visit her constituency in the diamond fields. On a subsequent visit to that country, to look at progress in maternal and reproductive health, we were shown around the parliament building by a lady who turned out to be her niece and put me in touch with the family, which was such a happy coincidence.

I was dispatched to Ghana a couple of months later to look at how water installations, paid for by the UK, were being cared for and used and finding a still chronic shortage of clean water in an African country that was considered to be doing well. It was a boring visit, made worse by two Californian academics who came with us and who had never been outside California before, let alone America. I think they got their passports, especially for the trip. The ignorance of the rest of the world in the USA is unbelievable, and yet they willingly support the military adventures of their President, who has not travelled much either.

Back home, my constituency at that time was getting more and more concerned about the prospect of a third runway at Heathrow, and a petition was being launched across west London by MPs concerned for the sanity of their constituents, John McDonnell, Labour MP for Hayes and Harlington, now Shadow Chancellor, being one of them. Ed Davey, MP for Kingston, and I were fighting another battle with the new breed of health service bureaucrats who were trying to remove the excellent John Langhan, Chief Executive at Kingston Hospital. He had grown up through the ranks and knew his job superbly, but was resisting the new wave of managers who talk about 'going forward' and 'patient journeys' and thought they were the bee's knees in healthcare when a lot of them had never seen a patient in their lives. We lost the battle, and John went on to other things, to our hospital's loss. That is progress.

It was time to return to Africa and receive an antidote to Sierra Leone. Two of us were invited by the Botswana High Commission to visit that country so that we could look at the problems it had. Botswana is the success story of Africa. It gained independence in

1966, the capital was moved to Gaborone and, with Seretse Khama as its president, the country went from strength to strength. At the time of independence, diamonds had been discovered in the north of the country by De Beers and, fearful of the corruption and exploitation that had happened in Sierra Leone, the president and De Beers came to an agreement that the proceeds of the diamond sales would be shared equally between De Beers and Botswana and the whole process would be continually monitored for corruption. Seretse Khama and his English wife Ruth made sure that the people benefitted from the diamond revenue and that workers for De Beers had good conditions. De Beers even made sure, when the AIDS crisis erupted, that workers in their mines were employed on condition that they attended for tests and treatment as that came online. Consequently, even though Seretse Khama died and his son was elected president, Botswana remains top of Transparency International's tables for no corruption.

We were introduced to other problems coming down the line, though. The first was to have second thoughts about elephant conservation. Everyone, including me, loves elephants. They are wonderful creatures and endangered in many parts of Africa because of ivory poaching. In Botswana, however, there is little poaching because of good management of the game areas, and the elephants were running amok through the countryside, damaging vegetation wherever they went and making life very precarious for other animals, such as giraffes which were under threat. A similar but human situation had developed in the Kalahari Desert where the Bushmen have traditionally roamed, and which the government was hoping to utilise as part game park for tourists, with the bushmen acting as wardens if they would live in settled villages built for them around the park. They had also started to use guns instead of bows and arrows to kill animals, and this was a threat to the very wildlife the government wished to conserve. Needless to say, there were other complicating factors, such as part of the Kalahari having diamonds, and permits to mine there had been given. Survival International predictably had started a campaign to save the Bushmen, but after seeing the life that they were living and what was on offer from the government, it became very difficult to take sides. It illustrated the dilemmas of development and how to improve people's lives in the nation as a whole, versus the needs of groups like the Bushmen, who generate such emotion in the West. It is a huge problem. Botswana is trying.

After a follow-up visit to Rwanda, it was conferences in Ottawa and meetings with the great Dr Seth Berkley of the International AIDS Vaccine Initiative. As 2002 drew to its close, the drums of war were beating again. Afghanistan had been forgotten, although the war was still raging there and people were dying in thousands, and George Bush wanted support for an invasion of Iraq, where the ghastly Saddam Hussein was accused by the Americans of having weapons of mass destruction and also of harbouring Osama bin Laden.

Chapter 18: Drums of War

The run-up to the Iraq War was the most terrifying thing I had experienced in parliament up to then. Seemingly rational people who had done some good things since taking office, Tony Blair, in particular, seemed to my medical eye to be completely besotted by George Bush and ready to follow him anywhere. Bush clearly wanted to make war on Iraq. The real reason was not clear, but war is good business in America, and they seldom reap the consequences as a nation so they can be excused for wanting to boost the American economy. That may seem harsh and too simplistic, but there was no logical reason for invading Iraq as there had been in George Bush's father's day when Saddam had invaded Kuwait.

International inspectors from the International Atomic Energy Agency, led by Hans Blix, had been sent out to Iraq and were allowed access to all the potential sites: they found no weapons of mass destruction, which were being used as the excuse for war. Bush and Blair met at Camp David for 'talks', but it is difficult to forget those swaggering pictures of Blair, thumbs tucked into the pockets of his jeans, striding proudly beside George Bush, his hero. Why, oh why, was Blair like this? Was it his successes in Sierra Leone and Kosovo and the adulation he received for those actions that made him love the thought of more glory? I was reminded of those children of huntsmen who are smeared with the fox's blood after their first meet to ensure their love of fox hunting thereafter. Had Blair been smeared with blood, or was he just flattered to be the friend of an American President? Whatever the reason, Parliament was going to approve. The Labour Party, with the exception of Jeremy Corbyn and John McDonnell, supported Blair. The whole of the Conservative party, except for Ken Clarke, was also ready to back Blair. So it seemed was my party, the Liberal Democrats, overwhelmingly male and scenting action as men do. Ming Campbell, our foreign affairs spokesman, was ill at the time but was insisting that a vote at the United Nations was necessary before Iraq could be invaded. UN Resolution 1441 had warned Iraq of serious consequences for non-compliance with the inspectors but had not authorised war. Despite this, and without Ming to hold them back, the foreign affairs team was very gung-ho and were pushing the party to support Blair.

Evidence had been produced to back up the claim that Saddam had weapons of mass destruction in the form of two 'dossiers' of evidence, the second of which was published in late January. Before I went into the party meeting one January afternoon, I went into the library of the House of Commons and asked if they had a copy of the second paper or 'dossier of evidence' produced by the government. I was handed this very 'dodgy' looking dossier, stapled together like someone's project for an exam. I simply could not believe it. Saddam, it was said, had weapons that could reach us in 45 minutes! This was backed by very amateur looking sketches and rubbishy text which said very little. Who was I to blow against the wind? I decided to try, even though I knew that as a mere woman, the men would try to shout me down.

I stormed into the party meeting, where they were nodding sagely about the need to go to war and all looking pretty excited about it. I waved the dossier in the air and said this was no better than an A-Level paper produced by a student, and we were being duped. We could not possibly go to war on this evidence. There were scandalised remarks. Who was this, a mere woman, daring to question the wise judgement of a bunch of men, most of whom had never been into a war zone or a famine-stricken area as I had and were simply doing what men do? Charles Kennedy, to do him justice, looked doubtful but said nothing, wisely waiting to hear what the majority said. Ming Campbell, who may have introduced a sane legal view, was ill and not present. When I was at my most embattled, Shirley Williams walked in. She agreed with me and argued in a very coherent way, as only Shirley can, that we could not support this without a second UN Resolution. The party broke up, and Charles decided we should oppose the war in the absence of a second UN resolution. I opposed the war with no conditions.

War solves nothing. The battle then was on to get Charles to go public in a big way.

Kate Hudson of CND was one of the leaders of the Stop the War Campaign, and a big anti-war rally was organised for Saturday, 15 February 2003. People were being encouraged to march and assemble for the rally in Hyde Park, where there would be speakers from every party. Kate asked me to try to persuade Charles Kennedy to speak for the LibDems. He was proving very reluctant, but she asked me to keep trying and got me to agree to be there to speak for the LibDems if he continued to refuse. I contacted Charles' office every day in the run-up to that rally and thought by the evening before that he was not going to do it. So I rang the CND office and asked when and where they wanted me to appear. To my delight and astonishment, they said Charles had agreed at the last minute and would be there. My delight was tinged with irritation that nobody in Charles' office had bothered to tell me, and my irritation increased the next day to find that I was ignored by the platform party before the march set off, with all the usual male sycophants dough-nutting around Charles like they had been born opposing wars. What hypocrites.

That day was the greatest show of opposition to a government's proposed action in our history up to then. Over a million people marched in central London, and all over the country, there were similar demonstrations, with huge numbers turning out on that bitterly cold February day. It was echoed all over the world, with every major city experiencing anti-war demonstrations. A great day for ordinary people and a shameful day for the leaders of America and the United Kingdom. I had to content myself with the knowledge that I had played a small part in getting my party to do the right thing. LibDem politicians still proudly boast how the party opposed the Iraq War.

A few days later, Robin Cook resigned as Foreign Secretary in one of those speeches in the House of Commons, which will go down in history. The famous 'Dodgy Dossier' was indeed shown to be the work of a Californian student by the name of Ibrahim al-Marashi, who had no idea that his musings about Iraq had been seen by civil servants in the Foreign Office and used and altered without his permission, but presumably with the knowledge of government advisors, to make the case for war. The Chilcot Inquiry revealed all eventually, but our leaders at that time have escaped censure somehow, despite rumblings on social media about war criminals and the International Criminal Court. Nevertheless, Iraq was invaded, and the Middle East was set on fire. That fire has spread and is still raging.

I think that this episode sowed doubts in my mind about whether I should carry on in parliament and for how long. I felt lost in that fog, like the engine smoke that used to envelope me as a child, but instead of imagining wonderful and exciting futures for myself, all I could see was confusion and having to put up with boneheaded politicians. Did I want to carry on indefinitely, being teased about being the Mother Teresa of the party? Would anyone ever link war with poverty or recognise it is in our interest as well as that of the people in developing countries to give them aid? We need to concentrate on women too, to give them the chance to be part of their country and not just baby machines until they die. 'Empowerment' was a popular word, but not very popular in governments, or my political party, at that time. Women in developing countries cannot be empowered until they have power over their own bodies and the ability to choose how many children they have. I make no apology for repeating that sentence over and over again. Why could other politicians not see the links?

Overseas aid had become one of my passions, but it entailed huge amounts of travelling all over the world, and I received hardly any recognition for what I was doing. I had been recognised as a trouble-maker, and therefore I should be kept busy. Charles Kennedy certainly had no interest in giving me another brief, so I rumbled on, wanting to spend more time in Richmond and with my family. My husband, who was also my best friend, had had a quadruple coronary bypass eight years before, and I think he wanted me to be around a bit more. He was such a tolerant and supportive man, but he had, after all, married a fellow medic and had every right to expect a bit more company.

Nevertheless, 2003 carried on, and a visit to Malawi had been scheduled to look at maternal health and DFID projects there. Malawi is a beautiful country, as are many African countries, but cursed by poverty, rotten government and corruption. It was the first country I had visited where we saw the ravages of the AIDS epidemic sweeping across Africa. The District Hospital in Blantyre was unbelievable. The wards were full of patients who shared beds, taking it in turns to lie down. They all had AIDS. There was no treatment then except to try to alleviate the suffering and rehydrate them. There were patients in the corridors and the hospital grounds outside. There were patients everywhere, desperate, dying people.

It was in Malawi that I heard the story of the Catholic bishop, who in response to his religious superiors' refusal to accept the use of condoms or any form of contraception, except the so-called 'safe' period, nevertheless helped the battle against the AIDS epidemic by saying, 'A man who knows he has AIDS, who has sexual intercourse without wearing a condom, is effectively committing murder. A woman who has sexual intercourse with a man, without establishing first whether he has AIDS or not, is effectively committing suicide. Both murder and suicide are sins in the eyes of God; therefore, to have sexual intercourse without using condoms is a sin in the eyes of God.' I wish I could have met that man.

With no medical care anywhere except in hospitals, the relatives of sick people simply brought them to the hospital and left them. The staff there were acting as mortuary attendants in many cases, receiving people into a ward and then shipping them out a few days later when they had died. The few trained doctors and nurses there, who could have relieved the pressure on hospitals, were leaving in droves to go to better working conditions in South Africa and some to Europe. We talked to a brilliant young woman doctor who was trying to persuade her seniors to set up mobile health care units to go round the countryside to try to treat and advise families with sick members to stay where they were. There also needed to be much more emphasis on the prevention of this disease which disproportionately affects more women than men because of the mode of transmission through body fluids. Tragically too, babies can contract AIDS at birth from their mothers or during breastfeeding. This was a few years before the introduction first of drugs that would stop transmission from mother to baby, and then the antiretroviral drugs, which have finally controlled the disease and given AIDS victims their lives back. I have not been back to Malawi but would love to see how that hospital is now – transformed, I hope, and success for that young doctor who wanted to introduce health teams for the countryside. I do know there is a link now with St Andrews University in Scotland.

Towards the end of the year, the LibDems won a by-election in Brent, and I was thrilled to introduce Sarah Teather MP into the House of Commons. She was a brilliant MP, but I suspect she had the same feelings as me about the place.

On Boxing Day 2003, our fifth grandchild was born. What a Christmas!

Chapter 19: The Unholy Land

Early in 2004, a year which was to prove a turning point in my life in several ways, I was asked to speak at a meeting of the Palestine Solidarity Campaign alongside the Palestinian Ambassador, Afif Safieh. Our government still refuses to recognise Palestine as a state, so it insists on calling the embassy a 'mission'. Nevertheless, most of us call an ambassador an ambassador when we see one, especially if he/she is Palestinian. I was asked because the previous year, I had been taken to Israel and Palestine with Oona King. It was not strictly a developing country, and I had had little contact with the subject because it was regarded as part of the foreign affairs brief. I had, however, deputised for Ming Campbell during a debate on the Middle East and took the usual 'balanced approach' required by Ming and the party. I shudder when I think of my ignorance on that occasion and apologise to any supporter of the Palestinian cause for making such spineless comments then. Before I left for my trip to Israel and Palestine, I was telephoned by a member of LibDem Friends of Israel to try to persuade me not to go with Christian Aid, who might give me a biased view but to wait until I could go on a trip sponsored by Friends of Israel, which would be more balanced and could offer much better accommodation and experience. Looking back on what has happened since then, I can smile.

Oona's mother was Jewish and unhappy about the then Israeli government's treatment of Palestinians, so Oona was extremely enthusiastic to see what was happening there. We went along with our 'minder' William Bell of Christian Aid, who was extremely concerned about deteriorating conditions for people in the West Bank and Gaza, and a second uprising called 'Intifada' had begun. The Palestinians were using suicide bombers going into Israel in protest. A ghastly development and a sad outlet for the desperation felt by young Palestinians.

Israel was allowing 'settlements' to be built in the West Bank, which was designated for the future Palestinian state. The word 'settlement' sounds innocent enough, but they were towns with town centres and public buildings and schools. Oona and I stood on a platform in one settlement with Jeff Halper of the Israel Committee Against House Demolitions (ICAHD) and heard him describe what he thought was his government's plan. The West Bank would be progressively built upon, with settlements connected by roads that only Israelis could use, cutting Palestinians off from each other's towns and villages and making what used to be a short journey into hours-long journeys as they navigated around the roads and new Israeli townships. A 'Swiss Cheese' of a country is how Jeff described it. Full of holes. To make matters worse, the houses were very different from the traditional smaller houses lived in by Palestinians and had reliable power and water supplies. The drainage and sewage were, in some cases, allowed to drain away onto Palestinian lands.

I remember one day driving out of Bethlehem after hearing that the houses there got clean water through their taps about twice a week if they were lucky, and noticing, as we approached a new settlement just outside Jerusalem, that there were sprinklers on the lawns. Precious water from the Palestinian hills being used to keep grass green in private Israeli gardens! There is now a serious concern for water supplies in Palestine and its neighbours, Jordan and Syria because Israel has nearly drained the River Jordan dry, and the Sea of Galilee is at seriously low levels. In recompense, brilliant Israeli engineers and scientists are desalinating seawater to ensure a supply for Israelis.

A visit to pay our respects to Yasser Arafat had been arranged, and we set off one morning to his blockaded compound, heavily guarded and with sandbags inside and out. We were met at the gate of this curious complex by soldiers and escorted through dark passageways, past more soldiers and groups of men just standing around and smoking. Everyone smoked. The air was thick and choking. We were ushered into a room with a long table surrounded by more men, all smoking, at the head of which sat Yasser Arafat, looking just like his photographs, although I noticed, very cyanosed and wheezing. Hanan Ashwari, the only woman in the room, sat beside him, feeding him from time to time with pills. I wondered then just how ill this man was, but he greeted Oona and me warmly with kisses, starting at the wrist and continuing upwards. He seemed genuinely pleased to see UK parliamentarians. The 'conversation' we were expecting turned out to be a very long, impassioned speech starting with the Balfour Declaration and continuing with every insult and betrayal perpetrated on the Palestinian people up to the time of our visit. We departed feeling suitably chastised.

No progress had been made after the much-lauded 'Oslo Accord' in 1993 when Arafat and Prime Minister of Israel Yitzhak Rabin had been awarded the Nobel Peace Prize. Everything had got steadily worse: the peacemaker Rabin was assassinated by an extremist Zionist, and the Israeli government just carried on with its expansion into the West Bank in total defiance of the agreement.

The occupying Israel Defense Forces, the IDF, made life frustrating and difficult for everyone, with random checkpoints to inspect papers and raids on Palestinian homes in the middle of the night to check there were no 'terrorists' hiding. Children were routinely roughed up on their way to school and sometimes arrested for alleged stone-throwing. We learned how children were tried in courts without a parent present and where only Hebrew was spoken. They were made to sign statements written in Hebrew, under extreme duress, and at all times treated with brutality. Some years after our visit, a group of lawyers led by Baroness Scotland, herself an eminent lawyer, produced a damning report entitled 'Children in Military Custody', but no action was taken or expected by our government.

It was so ironic that the Israelis were always accusing Palestinians of teaching hatred of Israelis in their schools—no need to teach hatred. The children couldn't but help but hate Israelis with the treatment they were getting. Olive groves were being torched and crops destroyed, and what produce the Palestinian farmers managed to grow often rotted because of delays imposed at the checkpoints. I have never forgotten an incident at a checkpoint when we were stopped, and 'papers' were demanded from our Arab Israeli driver. He duly handed them over, and the guard walked away. Some half an hour later, he returned with a swagger and pushed them towards our driver. As our driver reached for them, the guard threw them on the ground in disdain and walked away, leaving our driver to jump out and scrabble about in the dust and wind to gather up his precious identity, without which he could not work. He told us it often happened—routine treatment.

The checkpoint at the Erez Crossing into Gaza was particularly difficult. Gaza was regarded with great suspicion because some of the Hamas leaders were there, and Gaza was effectively ruled by them, a relatively new development in embattled Palestine. Palestinians who had become frustrated with the leadership of Yasser Arafat had, with the Israeli government's encouragement, formed a new Islamic style movement called Hamas. They were becoming increasingly popular with ordinary Palestinians. A faction called Islamic Jihad was there too, who fired homemade rockets sporadically into less populated parts of southern Israel.

At the Erez checkpoint, we met a woman who had been waiting two days to take her tomatoes to sell in Gaza, but they were ripening so fast in the heat that they would not be much good. This was a regular occurrence. At the same checkpoint, I must recall, Oona was desperate to go to the loo and asked permission from a soldier. He laughed and pointed to the bushes, where women were expected to go. Fine for a liberated western woman like Oona, but shaming for a much more modest Palestinian woman who sometimes also faced strip-searching at the checkpoints. Gaza was under strict military control and living under much worse conditions even than the West Bank, and Oona, quite rightly, called it a 'ghetto' in an article she wrote whilst we were there. One day during our visit, while we were looking at plans for an agricultural project being funded by DFID, a rocket suddenly flew over our heads, and we were ordered to get under the table in case of Israeli reprisals. The home-made rocket had been fired in response to an attack by helicopter guns on a car in central Gaza City, carrying Dr Rantisi, a prominent member of Hamas and a paediatrician. He was not killed, only wounded on that occasion, but was assassinated some months later by another Israeli attack. Such was life in Gaza.

There were no suicide bombings during our stay, but they had become almost the only way the Palestinians could think of to resist. By persuading fanatical, despairing, angry young people that their reward would be in paradise, young men and women were blowing themselves up in public places in Israel if they could get through the barriers and checkpoints. There were many deaths and injuries. I wondered how they could be so brave and yet so cruel. Hatred breeds violence.

I visited a clinic where women diagnosed with breast cancer could not hold out much hope of treatment unless they could afford expensive therapies in one of the big hospitals in Israel, which required long waits to get visas. We heard stories of women with obstetric complications dying with their newborn babies at checkpoints in the wait to get through. Surely I thought, if a country was occupying another, they should be responsible for public services to the occupied people. But of course, the Israeli government regards the whole of Palestine as their God-given land and therefore, the Palestinian people have no right to be there, even if they had lived there for generations, unlike the immigrant Eastern European Zionists, many of whom had probably never had any connection with the land of Israel except their religion. Some of them have more claim to the Russian Steppes than they do to land in the Middle East. I met one soldier at this checkpoint who could speak a little English: he explained that he was Russian and had 'converted' to Judaism to get the better life offered by Israel.

If only the Balfour Declaration had not spurred them on to create a Jewish State and if only they had not forgotten the second half of that declaration which said that after 'viewing with favour the establishment of a national home for the Jewish people', it also said, 'it being clearly understood that nothing shall be done which may prejudice the civil and religious rights of existing non-Jewish communities in Palestine.' The Palestinians had at no stage been consulted. Immigrants had been coming in since long before the Holocaust, which had confirmed the need for a home for the Jews. You cannot blame the Palestinians for resisting the formation of this 'home' for the Jewish people. They have a right to self-defence. I had become more and more angry and disillusioned during that visit. This Holy Land I had learned about in my childhood was a ghastly place of misery and hardship and, more than anything else, *humiliation*.

The Palestinians were subjected to daily humiliation by Israeli officialdom. I had seen grinding poverty in the poorest parts of the world. I had seen cruelty and warfare inflicting such suffering on oppressed people, but I had never seen such active and intense humiliation of mothers, fathers and children in front of friends and family and with such ghastly disdain with the power imposed by the Israeli soldiers. I could write a separate book about conditions in Palestine and Gaza over the years I have visited, but many have already done this. There are countless books about the Palestinian resistance and the brutal attacks by Israel on them, which our media like to call 'wars'. They are not warring because Palestine has no army. They are attacks by strong and all-powerful Israel against defenceless Palestinians. I have a growing pile of books about Palestine and Israel beside my bed which is constantly being added to. I should be reading them all, I know, but a few visits there are much better lessons than books. Others have also written about the history of this outrage much more graphically than I ever could.

That first visit left a huge impression on Oona King and me and is why at a meeting in the House of Commons in early 2004, having described the conditions in Palestine, I struggled to find a final sentence that would hit home. I always identify with the women wherever I go, and the women of Palestine are heroines, coping with poor living conditions and constant harassment, and the frequent imprisonment and deaths of their children and husbands at the hands of the Israel Defence Forces. I said what I truly felt, and that was, 'If I had been a Palestinian grandmother, struggling to bring up her family in those conditions, I might have considered becoming a suicide bomber myself.' It seemed a reasonable statement at the time. It did not mean that I approved – I did not. It just meant that considering all the circumstances, I had enough empathy to understand why they did it, or in many cases, were encouraged to do it by their leaders at the time. The sky fell on my head, and a new phase of my life began.

I was telephoned the next day by Charles Kennedy and had the one and only conversation I ever had with that man because communication usually came from his secretary Anna Werrin. He said that I must apologise and withdraw my remarks. I responded that the remark was out there and had been truly felt and, if he did not understand, he should go out to see the situation for himself. He said if I did not apologise, it would damage the party, but I stuck to my line. I do not think I have ever been so angry and disgusted with the party hierarchy, for that is what it was. I later found out from a friendly 'mole' at party headquarters that a very large donation to the party was in jeopardy if I was not 'dealt with'. A head had to roll, and it was mine. It rolled onto the backbenches, where I received friendship and support from all sorts of MPs.

The next morning in the lift, I received a hug and a kiss and a 'well done' from a Tory MP I hardly knew then. I did not complain. I hope I encouraged many other MPs to go out there, not always sponsored by the Friends of Israel groups attached to each political party, which give so much support and five-star 'jollies' in Israel to their supporters. One person, in particular, crossed the floor of the house to sit and talk to me and empathise – it was Clare Short, who had resigned from the government after the Iraq war fiasco. She has since become a good friend and has always been a fellow supporter of justice for the Palestinian people. We became board members for several years of the Welfare Association UK, which is a Geneva-based charity dispensing aid to Palestinian refugees in Lebanon and the ever-growing number of Palestinians trapped in

Gaza.

I received well over a thousand emails and letters, which were about 70 per cent supportive. I had two volunteers in my office to help answer them. The non-supportive ones were a revelation. I had never received such imaginative, obscene threats in my whole time as an MP. MPs often get nasty letters from people who cannot think of a good argument to promote their cause, so they just abuse us. Nothing, however, compares to the imagery of drowning in pig shit and some very inventive sexual threats I received then. I must not repeat them. Do these people get some relief, mental or physical, by throwing out this abuse at people they do not know? I think they must, and one must feel sorry for them. It is very rare for someone actually to tackle you face to face.

The internet is wonderfully anonymous for abusers. I have had several such episodes since, but nothing quite compared with that one, and I think these insulting messages should be deleted and forgotten, lest by reacting, we encourage more. Others disagree and dwell on them. I do not. If people cannot stand the truth, then I feel sorry for them, and I will not encourage them by reacting to their filth. Quite a debate about my remark ensued on programmes like Any Questions and Question Time, and the personal abuse continued.

The BBC Today programme contacted me and asked if I would go out to Israel and the occupied territories with James Reynolds, their Middle East correspondent at the time, and make a series of reports for the programme to run for a week. The idea was for me to meet both the families of suicide bombers, their victims and the people who had to deal with the aftermath of each incident. The Today programme then planned an open phone line for people to ring in with their comments after each day's report, but it closed after a couple of days because the lines were jammed.

The trip lasted a week, and the producers of the programme declared that to ease my pain, I was to stay at the American Colony Hotel, which I already regarded as the most beautiful hotel in the world. It developed from a charitable operation set up by the Spafford family in 1881, who were devout Christians and decided to leave their home in Chicago and live in Jerusalem. As time passed, they needed bigger premises, and they bought a large pasha's palace, which became the American Colony Hotel. It is famous for several things apart from its beauty. It was used by the grandfather of Sir Peter Ustinov to accommodate his guests when they visited Jerusalem, and a white sheet was flown from its roof when the Ottoman Empire was finally defeated. It has been regarded as 'neutral' territory ever since. Perhaps of greatest delight to me is that a descendant of the Spafford family is married to a now-retired member of the House of Lords and still works hard to raise money for Palestinian charities, particularly encouraging young musicians. I had previously only been there for drinks in its glorious central courtyard. My room was ancient and beautiful too, and every morning I woke to the sound of the low, rumbling voice of the muezzin atop the minaret nearby calling us to prayer. There is nothing quite like that sound. It is the voice of the Middle East.

The families of suicide bombers had, on the whole, no idea that their children were going to do this terrible thing until they heard the news and were only consoled by the fact that their child would be in paradise. Religion has a lot to answer for, but in this particular circumstance, I saw how powerful it had become. Young people with not much hope for the future, often with higher education and university degrees, much encouraged in Palestinian society, were doing nothing. Some had poor jobs if they were lucky and more humiliation. They were persuaded to end their lives in a blaze of glory on their way, as martyrs, to paradise. For me, it represented a waste of idealistic young lives and innocent Israeli lives, but nevertheless, I understood and wondered just what I would have done in that situation. In Israel, the families of the victims were also a surprise. Many of them, whilst grieving terribly for their loved ones, nevertheless had some understanding of why it was happening. Some blamed the wicked ideology of the Palestinians and others the incompetence of the Israeli government, which was failing to protect them. No one seemed to appreciate the conditions in which Palestinians were living due to the occupation. Nobody ventured into the West Bank anyway. It was considered much too dangerous. At least Israeli citizens had the superb facilities at the Hadassah Hospital in Jerusalem to help those who survived a bombing, facilities which completely amazed me. They were far superior to anything we had in the UK.

One afternoon I was taken to Bethlehem to meet some al-Aqsa Brigade militants. The Israelis regard them as terrorists, but to Palestinians, they are freedom fighters. We were to go to a Christian house donated for the meeting on the edge of the area called Shepherds' Fields, where we have always been told the angels appeared long ago. On the way, we were held up by a huge funeral procession winding its way into Nativity Square of a young girl who had died from leukaemia – not a bombing. As I stood with James patiently waiting for the crowds to clear, I reflected on how the death of a young person seems so much more of a tragedy than that of an old person who has lived their life. I did not realise that day what a portent that funeral was. After standing in the cold and rain, watching the crowds gradually clear, and watching Israeli surveillance jets fly overhead, two bearded men with shades, and pistols at their hips, got out of a car and approached us, stopping to talk to people on the way. Rather comical, I thought, when this meeting was supposed to be very hushed up. We eventually met a guide who spirited us away to meet the masked fighters for al-Aqsa.

The venue was a rather suburban part of Bethlehem and did not fit my image of the legendary fields where the birth of Jesus was proclaimed to the shepherds. The house we entered was very near the chapel marking the spot and was lavishly furnished with deep sofas and rugs. On one sofa, with a huge picture of Jesus on the wall behind, sat two heavily armed and masked men, members of the al-Aqsa Brigade. It was interesting to be told that the al-Aqsa Brigade had Christian and Muslim members. The conversation was about their justification for fighting the occupation, the injustice of the situation in which the Palestinian people found themselves, and that the UK was mainly responsible for their plight, which has been true, ever since that Sykes-Picot Agreement, followed by the Balfour Declaration. They spent most of the time we had with them berating western governments and saying that they would only accept Israel's right to exist if they got back to the borders set by the UN in 1947. Until then, they had a right to fight and defend themselves. In response to my plea not to use young people as suicide bombers, they said, 'We will not use them if you give us tanks and guns like the Israelis have. We use the resources we have.' Eventually, after sipping mint tea a little longer, we left the strange hornet's nest with Jesus on the wall and went back to Jerusalem and the haven of the American Colony Hotel, worlds away from the real Palestine. A rainbow appeared in the sky over the Holy City as we approached. A divine message of hope? I doubted it.

The next day, sitting in an office with some community leaders, a large ceremonial sword rattled on the wall and fell off. We were immediately ordered outside, where the earth shook a little more and then settled down. This was my first experience of an earthquake, apart from a 'pretend' one in a Japanese museum years before. For the rest of that day, wherever we went, families were living outside, presumably until they were sure no more shakes would disturb the peace.

At the end of that day, James took me to the road junction where the latest suicide bombing had taken place and asked me if I would still consider becoming a suicide bomber myself if I was Palestinian. I answered no, because I was simply not brave enough, had not enough religious faith, and was not living as Palestinians had to live, but after seeing and talking to families from both sides of the divide, I understood even better how it happened.

Thunder rumbled in the distance, warning me of the storms I would face in the years ahead for my support of these resilient people. I was to learn that any criticism of Israel or empathy with

Palestinians was to be greeted with a storm of abusive letters and phone calls and accusations of antisemitism, which no doubt were organised in some way. That brief remark about suicide bombers changed my life and my focus. I was suddenly in demand for all sorts of meetings and rallies and became a marching colleague of Jeremy Corbyn, who is a rare example of a totally honest and principled human being who fights for justice.

A delegation from the Palestinian Authority came over to the UK, and I was asked to entertain them for a day. I did so by taking them all to lunch and a brief tour of Kew Gardens, which in May is absolutely at its best. Comparisons kept being made with what they were going back to the next day. I felt mortified that all I could offer was a promise to continue to highlight the Palestinian cause whenever I could.

The only female member of the delegation unpinned a brooch from her dress and gave it to me. Made in Palestine – I still have it. Women politicians are very scarce in Palestine, as they are in many countries, and our own country does not set a particularly good example. Such a pity, I feel, when we are half of the population and are responsible for the nurturing of the next generation, a fact which seems to escape most men. This woman remarked that she wished Palestinian children had such a place to visit, free of soldiers and ugliness all around them.

I had to do some swift learning about Palestine. Being a medic and not a historian, I knew very little of the background to the situation, and people were always assuming that I did. History cannot be changed, and it has no bearing really on what goes on out there now. The Israelis claim it as their land, given to them by God, and one Zionist told me that their legal document is the Torah, which to the rest of us is part history and mostly myths and legends written down through the centuries. Hardly legally binding, but if so, why are the Ten Commandments not also legally binding: 'Thou shalt not kill.' 'Thou shalt not covet thy neighbour's house.' 'Thou shalt not steal.' Funny how obedience can be so selective sometimes. Leviticus is worth reading, too, for the laws it lays down. Do modern devout Zionists obey them all? Of course, they don't. For me, it is all about injustice, and that must be recognised and corrected.

My most memorable trips were to Gaza. An organisation called the European Campaign to End the Siege on Gaza wanted in 2008 to engage with politicians across Europe and to take them to Gaza to see conditions there. Gaza had been blockaded since 2006, and Israel controlled its borders. We had planned to go via Egypt, but at the last minute, we had been prevented by the Egyptians, so a linkage was made with the Free Gaza campaign, who were planning their second boat to sail there to 'Break the Siege'. This sounded all too exciting to miss, and so it was that we sailed on *Dignity.* A large pleasure cruiser, I suppose it was, but it only had one sleeping cabin, which Clare Short and I were allowed to use on the way back.

Onboard there were eleven parliamentarians from the UK, Ireland and the EU, including Clare, Lord Ahmed, and myself, plus over a ton of medical supplies. We left a Cypriot port to sail overnight to Gaza. Watching the sunset over the Mediterranean and sailing into the unknown was quite an experience and a bit daunting for me, who hates sailing, and resisted all attempts by my husband to get me sailing in his boat. He could hardly believe that I had consented. We were stopped by an Israeli gunboat as we approached Gazan waters, but when we gave the full list of passengers and an account of our cargo, we were allowed to pass – the last boat to be allowed - ever. After that, boats from the Free Gaza movement were boarded and taken to Israel, and the *Mavi Marmara* in 2010 was boarded by Israeli soldiers. Ten passengers were killed in the ensuing fight and several soldiers wounded. As usual, though, little was done, and Israel got away without censure.

As we approached Gaza Port, hundreds of little boats came sailing out to meet us. Waving flags and cheering, they escorted us into the harbour. It was such a unique and emotional moment, with many tears of joy being shed by Gazans and European parliamentarians alike. We did the usual round of meetings and inspections of schools, hospitals and infrastructure, all in poor condition due to a lack of materials to repair them. Israel forbids many raw materials to enter Gaza because they allege they could be used for making escape tunnels and rockets. On the voyage back, I watched dolphins beside the boat and what I think were flying fishes. As dawn was breaking, I sat in the prow of the boat, watching the sunrise as two of my colleagues challenged my agnosticism and tried to convert me to Islam. I would not be moved. If God exists, he has an awful lot to answer for, but the sunrise was spectacular! We did not know it then, but at the end of that year, the Israelis launched their most brutal attack so far on Gaza. It was called Operation Cast Lead and destroyed much of the infrastructure of Gaza and killed 1400 Gazans, and maimed thousands more.

Keith joined me on the next visit nearly two years after this horrible assault on innocent people, and this time the Egyptians allowed us in and gave permission, with dire warnings of being ambushed by terrorists, to cross the Sinai Desert in an old coach that we had hired. It was as great an experience as crossing the Med – even greater because I had never experienced the desert before, which is so beautiful in its way. Keith was remembering childhood years in Iraq and loving every moment. It was a long and hard journey and a relief once more to arrive in Gaza once we had been 'processed' by the officials at the Rafah Crossing. We were there, ready to see the carnage remaining after Operation Cast Lead. Schools destroyed. Hospitals badly damaged. Sewage flowing in some streets, and the sea was smelling of it. Amputees seemed to be everywhere. Nevertheless, Gazans as ever had retained their hope for the future, their resilience, and above all, their sense of humour. I sat on a bench one morning with an old man who remembered the British rule in Palestine and spoke some English. We were chatting about the future when suddenly we saw a heavily laden cart pass by pulled by a donkey. 'Look,' he said, 'my new Mercedes.' Chuckle.

On that visit, we saw some French archaeologists excavating the remains of an ancient monastery, which they said could be a great tourist attraction amongst others in the coastal haven that Gaza would become one day. I do not know if the archaeologists are still there or whether the remains of that old monastery is there. I do hope so.

In 2014 the Israelis launched an even deadlier attack on Gaza and killed over 2000 people, many of them children. More of Gaza was reduced to rubble. All done on some fabricated pretext or other about the 'threat' from the tunnels which the Gazans persisted in digging to smuggle in supplies and to try to escape. My uncle helped dig a tunnel out of the German prison camp, Stalag Luft 3, during the Second World War. Prisoners try to escape. The people of Gaza are no different, and the weapons they may have smuggled in are hardly a match for Israel which has one of the biggest armed forces in the world *and* nuclear weapons.

Since then, the cruelty of the Israeli Defence Force (IDF) towards the young people of Gaza has escalated, and at peaceful demonstrations, over this last year, they have killed many youngsters throwing stones from hundreds of yards away, and in particular, shooting young boys and men in the legs. Their injuries are so severe that despite the heroic efforts of surgeons working in poorly equipped hospitals in Gaza, provided by NGOs such as Medical Aid for Palestine and bolstered by visits from surgeons and physicians from Europe, many limbs are amputated. There are thousands of young amputees in Gaza now, with their lives and dreams ruined. I simply cannot describe the disgust I feel for the actions of the Israeli government, which remains our special friend and trading partner. I have no wish, either, to sound patronising, but the determination of Palestinians never to lose hope and to stay positive just amazes and impresses me. What also impresses me and depresses me at the same time is that they have large families, determined to hold onto their land with sheer numbers if need be. The women in the refugee camps all over the Middle East have the same attitude. A child killed means they should provide a replacement. It is also noteworthy that the Zionist settlers have large families, perhaps for the same reason? These often brutal and arrogant people, from anywhere but Palestine, now number over half a million in the West Bank, and they are gradually eating up what is left of the West Bank.

Before he left England, a Palestinian friend arranged many visits to encourage parliamentarians in Europe to engage more with the Palestinian cause. He was so energetic, and it was almost impossible to say no to him. We visited Damascus on three occasions: the first two were to meet the Hamas leader Khaled M'ashal and the President of Syria, Bashir Assad, who at that time was regarded fairly well by the West. He had been extremely welcoming to Palestinian refugees throughout the Iraq war and the continuing expulsion of Palestinians from their own lands. Both men were impressive, M'ashal in particular. He asked which Israel he was supposed to recognise and where its boundaries lay? A fair point, we thought. Since the 1967 war, nobody knows what the boundaries of Israel are, so how can they be recognised?

President Assad was tall, cultured, and spoke perfect English. Keith had known him when he worked at the Western Eye Hospital in London. Keith was a neuroradiologist, and Assad came over to St Thomas' to join Keith's ward rounds. I chatted to him about that. Such a polite and amiable man who has apparently turned into a monster over the last five years. What on earth happened to his Hippocratic oath, 'First do no harm'? The last time we met him was to plead on behalf of Palestinians trapped in a camp in the desert on the Iraqi border. We had visited them before we saw Assad. It was a well-run camp overseen by UNHCR, but the people wanted a proper life with access to a town or city. They were surrounded by desert – it had taken us seven long and hazardous hours to reach them by car. They had settled in Iraq after the Nakba when the state of Israel was created and had to flee for their lives. They had been made welcome in Iraq under Saddam Hussein and had now been driven from Iraq by the new government there, installed by the Americans and us. The new government was Shia; the

Palestinians are Sunni and so had to leave yet again. Assad was reluctant to take any more refugees.

Yarmouk camp in Damascus, which we had also visited, was well organised, and the people there had full access to Syrian schools and health facilities, but Assad did not want to take any more refugees without funding from the international community. He had enough problems feeding his own people. In the end, UNHCR managed to disperse the people in the desert camp all over the world to countries that would take them. ISIS infiltrated Syria and took over Yarmouk camp, which Assad then had an excuse to attack.

I visited Palestine again on many occasions until the Israeli authorities began stopping anyone going through Tel Aviv airport who was connected with the BDS (Boycott Divestment and Sanctions) campaign, which continues to gain support in much the same way as we exerted pressure on the South African government about apartheid. Fortunately, nowadays, with the internet and social media, we are all in hourly contact with friends and colleagues in the West Bank and Gaza. The Israelis have not blocked that – yet. In the following months and years, I made many speeches about Palestine and did many interviews. I was targeted by the Zionist press and media, who combed through every word I uttered to see if they could go on the attack.

Several more episodes are worth recording. During the ensuing election campaign in 2005, I was asked what I thought of a report in a Palestinian online 'newspaper' of which I was a patron. In that journal, it was reported that an American professor was alleging that the IDF disaster relief team was harvesting organs from the dead bodies in the Haitian earthquake. I responded by congratulating the IDF on their swift and efficient response to the disaster in Haiti and added that if there were any worries on that score, they should launch an inquiry to establish the truth. The next day the Jewish Chronicle was accusing me of 'blood libel', which was just about the most far-fetched and ridiculous thing I had ever heard. How can an inquiry to establish the truth be blood libel, and what self-respecting doctor like me would ever think it feasible to harvest organs from earthquake victims anyway? What utter nonsense, but I was again disciplined, and the officers of the party sent a letter to all candidates in the election, telling them to denounce me and what I was alleged to have said. My loyal doctor husband refused to let me do any more campaigning in the election and cancelled his (generous) subscription to the party. He never forgot that incident. He regarded it as an insult to our profession. The LibDem party officials were lucky to escape an action for libel against me, brought by my husband.

On another occasion, I was sent a copy of a book by Professors John Mearsheimer and Stephen Walt called *The Israel Lobby*. It was a brilliantly researched and authoritative book about the influence of an organisation called AIPAC, which stands for the American Israel Public Affairs Committee. It exists to promote the interests of the State of Israel and supports American politicians with huge amounts of money raised by its members, such as Sheldon Adelson, a great supporter of the government of Israel, who had made his billions in casinos. He was very close to Donald Trump, the recent occupant of the White House. The book revealed how much money poured into the coffers of the Republicans and the Democrats if they supported the government of Israel and anyone who did not had a very tough time of it at campaign time. The book caused great offence and was deemed to be antisemitic. The two professors had to leave the Kennedy School at Harvard University because the school, I was told, had lost so much donor money. What the book had said was shown to be true. The Israel Lobby was running America. The gun lobby indulges in similar activities, but they are home-grown. They do not represent a foreign power. Israel is the Promised Land for many Christian Evangelicals in America, too, looking forward to Armageddon and the Second Coming. They also have tremendous power over politicians in the USA. After my experience with my own party, I was constantly wondering if the same influences applied to our political parties and politicians. In the absence of public funding for political parties, it is inevitable that strong and rich lobby groups will influence our national life.

At a party gathering soon after the publication of Walt and Mearsheimer's book, I remarked that the Israel Lobby seemed to have its grips on the Western World – its financial grip. Under my breath, to a colleague, I added that after my experiences, I wondered if it had a grip on my party too. It was overheard, of course, and another storm ensued. Ming Campbell, then Leader of the Liberal Democrats, was obliged to discipline me, although I cannot remember how. He did make me agree, however, that considering what Hitler had accused the Jews of, it was a pretty incendiary remark to make, and I agreed on that occasion. However, having seen the influences on American politics and watching party antics carefully over the years culminating in a brilliant exposé of the Israeli Embassy activities in our parliament by a programme screened some years ago by Al Jazeera, I am sure I am right. The only answer is to limit election expenditure and the money spent on extra help in MPs' offices and have government funding of political parties. That is not popular with the voters, so it will not happen. We shall go on having governments influenced by outside lobbies.

On another occasion, I was asked to speak at Middlesex University at a meeting about Palestine, and my husband Keith, who had recently been with me on a trip to Jerusalem and Bethlehem, came with me. We had been on a short trip, self-funded, to celebrate my birthday in February, to see some projects being funded by the Welfare Association UK, a charity founded and largely funded by the Palestinian diaspora in the UK, led by the Qattan Foundation. One project was the restoration of the old pilgrims' quarters around the al-Aqsa mosque in Jerusalem, and we were privileged to be allowed onto that sacred mount, also known around the world as Temple Mount or the Dome of the Rock. We had walked the Via Dolorosa and purchased a chess set from a dusty shop in the old city. Keith was disgusted by the noise and crowds in the Church of the Holy Sepulchre, and, as I had struggled round it on a previous visit, we gave it a miss. One thing above all I loved about him was his absolute abhorrence of organised religion and the corruption it has spawned down the ages. It did not stop him from supporting our local parish church, St Anne's on Kew Green.

On my birthday, it was snowing hard, and Jerusalem had closed down, unused as they are to snow. We had been invited to lunch in Bethlehem by Samira Hassassian, the wife of the Palestinian Ambassador in London, and we desperately wanted to go to their family home in the hills overlooking Bethlehem. The hotel managed to find us a brave taxi driver who, with decent payment, offered to drive us there. So it was that we slowly crept by car and not by donkey, through the bleak midwinter over the Bethlehem hills to that little town. Samira insisted the taxi driver joined our lunch party, and we had a very merry time with a brief tour of Bethlehem thrown in. Samira was one of the loveliest, most generous and intelligent women I have ever met, but sadly she died not many years after this visit. On that trip, we treated ourselves by staying at the American Colony Hotel, which I had experienced with the BBC.

At Middlesex University, my fellow panellist was Ghada Karmi, my old medical colleague. Husband Keith decided to accompany me because having seen the situation for himself and loving the Middle East ever since he spent several years of his childhood in Iraq; he was getting more and more fired up about the situation and the regular attacks by the Israel Lobby on anyone who dared speak out against that government. He saw himself as my bodyguard, I think. I did not disappoint, and I made a remark pointing out that Israel could not continue in its present form unless it changed its policies towards the Palestinians and when the USA got tired of funding what I described as their aircraft carrier in the Middle East. The next day I was again summoned by my party leader, now Nick Clegg because the bloggers and the Jewish Chronicle were alleging that I was denying Israel's right to exist.

Very recently, I commented on social media that I wondered

whether the actions of the Israeli government towards the Palestinians were in any way responsible for the rise in antisemitism in Europe and the USA, a fact which seems patently obvious to me. Again I was attacked and denounced, my accusers saying that it was 'victim blame' and antisemitic to say such a thing. It is now antisemitic to say anything about the Israeli government, which can be twisted to mean criticism of the Jews. I never mention the Jewish diaspora. Why should I? They are not responsible for what the Israeli government does. I always direct my comments towards the Israeli government, but as Israel is now officially 'The Jewish State of Israel' and has a National State Law confirming the superiority of Jewish people in Israel, any criticism of the Jewish State government's policies is apparently antisemitic. It may seem convoluted, but it is taking hold. Even more worrying is President Macron of France declaring that anti-Zionism is antisemitic. Does that mean that criticising the Conservative and Unionist Party is anti-British?

The most serious and, in its way, ridiculous accusation came in 2016. I was asked by the Palestine Return Centre to host and chair a meeting in the House of Lords to herald the coming commemoration of the Balfour Declaration in 2017, for which many events and meetings were being planned. The very good speakers included Dr Ghada Karmi, Palestinian author of many books about her homeland and my old medical colleague, Karl Sabbagh, Palestinian author and Betty Hunter, Patron of the Palestine Solidarity Campaign. The meeting was packed and was also recorded by Al Jazeera, who had a press pass for the Palace of Westminster but had not obtained special permission to film this meeting, for which I was castigated. Although I had to apologise to the House authorities for this, it nevertheless proved very useful as events unfolded. During the meeting, a rabbi from Neturei Karta, a Haredim Jewish sect, went on a practically inaudible rant about some aspect of the problem, and I was glad when I heard him use the word 'sanction' and was able to stop him speaking and move the discussion on to considering the BDS movement, for which I was applauded by the audience. Neturei Karta is a colourful and friendly orthodox Jewish group that opposes the Jewish State of Israel and its government in particular. They want the old Palestine back, where all religions mixed freely and got on with their lives. They are implacably opposed to the Zionist movement.

I thought nothing more of this intervention until the next morning when, walking past the LibDem Whips' Office, I was called in to be told that I was suspended from the party pending an investigation into my chairing an antisemitic meeting in the House of Lords the previous evening. The national newspapers had received reports of this meeting, and I was castigated for encouraging antisemitic speech and applauding it afterwards. A Zionist blogger had been present at the meeting and had sent a report to the national newspapers about the rabbi's speech, alleging that he had talked about Hitler's friendship with the Zionist movement before the Second World War and that I had allowed loud applause for this speaker. This was untrue, and others confirmed at the meeting that nobody had heard exactly what this rabbi had said. The newspapers did not mention the fact that the speaker I allowed was a rabbi, albeit from a small sect detested by Zionists. Such is the trivia for which we are persecuted.

I was extremely angry and told the party that I was resigning there and then and that I refused to be treated in this way or 'investigated' and publicly castigated to the delight of my enemies. I have never rejoined the party which I had joined in 1959 and had worked for all my life. They are terrified of the Israel Lobby, like all political parties. A few individual politicians like me are not, thank goodness.

The House of Lords Commissioner was asked by the Board of Deputies of British Jews to investigate me, with a view to suspension from the House, and this was painstakingly done with interviews and statements over the next four months. The filming, which I had mistakenly allowed, was watched closely by the commissioner, who found nothing at the meeting to be antisemitic in any way. They accepted that hardly anybody could hear the rant and that the applause was not for the rant, but for me when I managed to move on and call another speaker, and that all I had said was, of course, true: a great relief after months of worry. Sadly, I have never received an apology for their poor judgment from the then leaders of the Liberal Democrat Party.

A week later, after a day of what felt like indigestion, I had a serious heart attack on the underground while on my way home in the evening. Was there any connection? We shall never know, but I am happy to say that John Lee, a Jewish peer, colleague and friend, hauled me off the train at never-to-be-forgotten Gloucester Road station, where the last thing I remember was looking up at its wonderful golden globe lights high above, appearing to move around like planets as I slipped in and out of consciousness. He called an ambulance, where I was resuscitated, stabilized, and taken eventually to the Hammersmith Hospital for stents to be inserted in my coronary arteries by a team led by Palestinian-born cardiologist Dr Ramzi Khamis.

I have never ceased to wonder at what seemed to be divine intervention, nor will I ever stop being grateful to that Jew and that Palestinian. I am a very fortunate woman. The 'enemy' on Facebook and the internet could not resist pointing out that my stents were probably made in Israel, and was I going to have them removed as I boycott goods and services from Israel? A quick phone call to my Palestinian cardiologist reassured me that he did not use Israeli-made stents, ever. Faith restored, I duly posted the news for all to read.

I have ploughed on, speaking all over the country when invited to do so and tabling questions to our government, drawing attention at every opportunity to the theft of land and the killing and maiming of the Palestinian people going on relentlessly in Palestine, ensuring that these atrocities are recorded in Hansard forever. The Israel Lobby, however, led by the Board of Deputies of British Jews and the Israeli Embassy, are now conducting a

McCarthy-like purge of all supporters of the Palestinian people, deeming it to be antisemitic. Attacks on Jeremy Corbyn, a lifelong supporter of justice and human rights, have been made for years, accusing him of antisemitism. Every remark anyone in public life makes about the injustices of the situation or that criticises the Israeli government is twisted into antisemitism in their judgement. This is so sad because I firmly contend that it is helping fuel the canker of antisemitism, not suppressing it.

Public meeting organisers and the owners of public halls are being targeted in a very frightening way if they dare to try to organise a meeting about Palestine. One meeting in Worthing two winters ago, which I spoke at with Tom Suarez, violinist and writer of books on Israel, had to move venue three times before it went ahead. Fortunately for us, the furore in the local press had brought in the crowds, and the hall we eventually landed up in was packed that night. Freedom of speech is being attacked in our universities and local communities, and no one seems to be concerned. Our government and its cowardly allies look on and express concern about Israel breaking International Law and making 'representations' to the Israeli government whilst protecting its financial interests and trade agreements by doing nothing.

Recently, a minister in the government of Israel, Ayelet Shaked, called for the destruction of Palestinian society and the slaughter of Palestinian mothers who give birth to little 'snakes'. This was not reported in our press: no fuss, no retraction, no request for an apology within Israel. They have freedom of speech there, it seems, but seek to curtail ours. What hypocrisy.

I get a great deal of support from many people, but it is mostly privately because of fear of attack, and if I ever say that I have Jewish friends who also support what I say and do, I am told I am dividing Jews into good and bad Jews, and that is antisemitic – work that one out? Nevertheless, our constant stream of questions to our government continues, and they will never be able to say that they did not know what was going on in the occupied territories of

Palestine. In the House of Lords, I have asked at least six questions each week about what is going on in the West Bank and Gaza, helped tremendously by my researchers and friends, Sally Fitzharris and Miranda Pinch. Miranda is of Jewish origin herself and has travelled extensively in Palestine. She has even made a film about the situation which she shows up and down the country. It is called 'From Balfour to Banksy', relating the changes in life in Palestine from the time of the Balfour Declaration to when the artist Banksy started doing his wonderful murals all over the separation wall that divides Israel and the West Bank, the most famous being of a little girl with a bunch of balloons floating upwards, hopefully towards freedom. He has also built a hotel abutting the wall, called the Walled-Off Hotel. A brilliant pun.

More recently, I have been horrified at the attacks on Jeremy Corbyn, accusing him of antisemitism and harbouring antisemites in the Labour Party, which led to the loss of confidence in that party during the General Election in December 2019. There was little discussion of the policies of that party, which for me were a refreshing return to the socialism of the Attlee government in the post-war years when I was a child. All the media could talk about was antisemitism, and I again got into trouble by pointing this out and making a flippant remark about Corbyn's enemies dancing in the streets when the Labour Party suffered a crushing defeat. I knew Jeremy well from years of campaigning for Palestine, and I also knew his Shadow Chancellor, John McDonnell, from campaigning against the expansion of Heathrow Airport – I had offered to lie down with Boris Johnson in front of bulldozers if the Third Runway went ahead. We have never been told what these incidents of antisemitism in the Labour Party were, beyond internet threats and abuse which I frequently receive. No other party was attacked or investigated in the same way. It was a direct attempt to discredit a good man who happened to promote left-wing policies alongside his support for human rights and international law. It was the most disgraceful episode in British politics.

I am also horrified by the meekness of some Palestine-supporting NGOs who stay quiet for fear of being accused of antisemitism. Why are they so timid? Is it because they fear for their jobs? They certainly have to fear for the safety of their organisations' bank accounts, which have been known to be frozen after accusations that the charity was helping terrorists, which is nonsense. The same accusation can be levelled at the Palestinian Authority and its leaders, who tiptoe around trying to stay as quiet as possible to preserve the lifestyle they enjoy on good salaries paid for by the international community. It highlights the question as to who is responsible for the costs of the occupation of Palestinian territory by Israel. According to International Law, it is the occupying power who should be paying the bill, but Israel has never been held to account on this matter. They get billions in aid from the USA to help subjugate the Palestinian people and the international community (mostly European countries), support the Palestinians. Is this legal or fair? I leave that question hanging there. Nevertheless, I will never give up on them. Whether I am in the House of Lords or not, questions will be tabled every week, putting on record the crimes of the occupation of Palestine and the callousness and cruelty of Israeli government agents. It will be a record for future generations to read and draw upon; as potent as any memorial, the record will be in Hansard forever.

But I must repeat over and over again: *I am not antisemitic. I have never been antisemitic. I will never be antisemitic.*

I am a campaigner for justice, and the Palestinians have suffered a terrible injustice for over a hundred years now, since the Balfour Declaration.

Chapter 20: Darkness

Back in 2004, I was looking forward to being out of Westminster, but I knew that the issue of Palestine would stay with me whatever I did in the future. I did finally confirm that I would stand down at the next election and do other things, like concentrating on my old speciality of women's health which was becoming so important in international development, campaigning for justice for Palestine, and rocking the cradles of grandchildren.

Susan Kramer was on the verge of being selected to take over from me: the stage was set for a different life, and I was beginning to enjoy the prospect of spending more time with my family. It is a boring old cliché, but you have to have been a member of parliament to understand just how little family life is possible whilst in the role. I used to try to insist with my team that Sunday should be mine, but it did not work out like that, and, having lived in the constituency for so long, every occasion was just an extension of the family with politics tagged on. By that time, too, I had five grandchildren with the prospect of more on the way!

Just after the summer session of 2004 ended, one brilliant sunny morning, I was tidying up and looking forward to my daughter, Mary, and her two little boys coming to stay for the weekend whilst her husband was working abroad. She had telephoned to say it would be around lunchtime, but mid-morning, we had a call from her husband, Jake, saying that just as he was boarding the plane, he had received a message to say that Mary was extremely ill and was on her way to hospital, the children being cared for by the kind neighbour who had found her. He was on his way back.

We drove as calmly as we could to the West Middlesex hospital, wondering all the way if the family curse of early death had visited our lovely daughter. We found her blue and lifeless, receiving treatment from an increasingly desperate team of doctors and nurses who it transpired had been using cardiopulmonary resuscitation for some long while, and we guessed they were waiting for her relatives to understand how hopeless the situation was. It was clear to her doctor parents that our only daughter was dead and not even the chance of a vegetable existence was there for her – not that we or anyone would have wanted that. Mary Louise was gone, and her two little boys, aged two and four, were motherless. Jake arrived, pale and shocked, and after saying our final goodbyes to Mary, we drove over to our grandchildren and took them home, where the rest of our two families and their friends gathered during the day to comfort each other. Our eldest grandson said that he had heard a shout whilst Mummy was emptying the dishwasher and found her lying 'asleep' on the floor. He could not wake her up, and he and his brother had started screaming and yelling. Their close friend and neighbour had heard the noise and came round to summon help. It was all too late.

It was not till later in the evening that we discovered that Mary had been the victim of a terrible accident. Many friends and family were gathered together in Mary's house that evening, and someone recalled that Mary had said there was 'static' coming from the utensil rack above the cooker. As far as I can remember, another family member must have summoned the police, because they arrived, together with an electrician who found that a live wire was in touch with screws holding that metal utensil rack because a cooker hood had been wrongly installed when the kitchen was refitted four years previously. The cable for the hood had been sunk into the plaster with no casing and had been stretched diagonally across the wall instead of horizontally and vertically, as is the rule. Over the years, the rack had sunk down slightly and was in touch with the unprotected wires of the cooker hood. Mary, holding the metal dishwasher door open with her ankle whilst hooking a metal spoon back on the rack, had completed the circuit, and she had been electrocuted. The post mortem confirmed this with the discovery of burns on her ankle.

Even now, after sixteen years, I find it difficult to recall that day, but I do remember that as crowds of their friends turned up to comfort my son-in-law, those two little boys became increasingly excited.

What goes through a child's mind on these occasions? I thought of the many orphan children I had seen all over the world in war zones; here we had our own war zone, with friends milling around, crying and grabbing each other.

Keith and I took our eldest grandson into the park to look for frogs, which he liked doing, and he was able to tell us on the way how he had tried to make Mummy better by getting a damp flannel for her head because that is what she did when he was poorly. He was anxious that he might have done the wrong thing. We reassured him, mentally noting how glad we were that Mary had been thrown away from contact with the metal before he did it; otherwise, he could have died too.

If there is one thing that immersion in international development issues has done for me, it is to realise what charmed lives we live here in the West. We comfort ourselves by contributing to charities working in war zones and after natural disasters and move on. Mothers die, often from complications of childbirth or during attacks on their homes and villages. Children die so often, and there are so many of them, that some people assume that perhaps it does not mean as much to lose a child in a large family as in our 'nuclear' families here.

Archbishop Tutu has reminded us that a mother grieves just as much for a dead child in a war zone as we do in privileged old England. I thought of that many times over the months following Mary's death and reminded myself that we had her two boys, still proof of a once-living and treasured daughter, and that those boys were everyone's priority now.

Mary's funeral in Richmond Parish Church was packed with friends and constituents and people who just knew our family and wanted to give us their support. I was taken back to Manger Square in Bethlehem when a year before, I had been caught up in a crowd moving into the Church of the Nativity following the bier of a young woman who had died in her prime. I am not a superstitious person, but in the heightened emotions of the time, it was difficult not to see it as some sort of omen. I resolved that day to watch over Mary's boys with the rest of the family, whilst never, ever, abandoning the cause of justice for Palestine, where so many young people are cut off in their prime by the actions of the Israel Defense Forces. Mary was the first person to ring me the morning after my 'suicide bomber' remark when the media was getting very excited. She had heard about it at the school gates and wanted me to know that she and her fellow mums understood the sentiment and were right with me.

As soon as I returned to Westminster, I was approached by a government minister who explained that the Labour government had been concerned for some time about electrical safety, which was not treated as seriously as safety for gas installations. They asked if I could bear to spearhead their campaign for what became known as 'Part P' of the Building Regulations, which required most electrical work to be done by a registered electrician or inspected by the local government building regulations people. It seemed like a good idea to me, and together with another family, whose mother had been electrocuted in her bath in a rented cottage because the water taps were live, we promoted the campaign and made films for the Electrical Safety Council, now called Electrical Safety First.

Interesting to note that amongst the mostly supportive letters, I got mail from amateur electricians who said I was putting them out of business and making them charge more for their work. Some letters were abusive. Some said my daughter's death was retribution for supporting the Palestinian people. One message of support for the family and me accused Mossad of killing my daughter, which actually made me laugh as the 'accident' had been set up by a careless electrician four years before Mary's death. It is always amazing to realise how many sick people there are out there, which is why my philosophy has always been 'delete and move on'. To respond to their abuse justifies it. They feel they have hit home and are making an impact. The only way to deal with it is to ignore it.

On the other hand, most of the messages we received after her death were comforting and moving. Gordon and Sarah Brown wrote to us, having experienced, two years before, the death of their tiny daughter a few days after her birth from a brain haemorrhage. I had been devastated for them both then. I was and still am a great fan of both Gordon and Sarah Brown. MPs who I had never spoken to before, including the Leader of the Opposition, Michael Howard, stopped and hugged me in the corridors of Westminster, and some shared their own experiences of the death of a child. Such humanity in such a usually combative place was so comforting. The other great comfort was how close I became to my daughters-in-law, and in particular, the youngest one, who I like to think has become my daughter too. Strange notions to be pondered at such times.

A few weeks later, I was invited by the Any Questions team onto their programme up in Ullapool, which provided a good excuse for Keith to join me afterwards, and we headed off in a hired car up the west coast, across the 'top' of Scotland, and down back to Inverness. I shall never forget the tranquillity and restorative powers of the lonely Scottish mountains and lakes. In the evening, when walking beside the Kyle of Tongue, there was a complete and very vivid rainbow over the hills. At times like that, you are susceptible to omens, and for me, that heralded comfort and optimism for the future of our family. To help me remember her and perhaps help others too, I wrote a poem about it. I found it very therapeutic, however bad the 'poetry' was, and recommend others in my situation to try the same thing. It helps keep the person alive.

To Mary Louise on Richmond Hill

Her laughter rings out still, my daughter remembered,
Fifteen long years since the laughter stopped, she died.
And yet I can still hear it loud and clear,
The lovely enlivening sound of a young woman in her prime.
She loved life did my daughter, squeezed it hard, drank

*every drop,
Never did things by halves, always full of ideas and adventure
For herself for her love, for her dear, dear children, her brothers,
But everything done with a sense of fun.
I remember her birth; swift, no messing, a brief hour of effort,
Then she was there, wrinkled face, screwed up eyes,
As I looked down at her, she seemed to be laughing even then,
Sorry I look such a fright, Mum, sorry if I was a pain!*

*And as this special girl grew up, she never gave up,
Loyal to her friends, to the exasperation of some others,
Poor grades, despair, then determination,
To show those pesky examiners her real mettle to succeed, which she did.
Never defeated, was she ever depressed? Always ready to defend the indefensible.*

*My daughter, killed by a careless electrician on a bad day
Not his fault, she would have said, we all have bad days.
My daughter, whose laughter I can still hear, ringing out.*

*I sit on the bench overlooking the best view in England, listening,
Where she spent evenings with the gang as a rebellious teenager,
Yes, getting cross with the anxious mother, when summoned to give the lift home,
Because it's a long walk and the bus has been missed.
As I sit on the bench, the laughter returns, and I think of her legacy,
Her two little boys, shocked and bewildered at first, but now,*

True to her genes, they laugh and have fun; perhaps they come here too,
And look to the bright future that she wanted for them.

I sit on the bench, and her laughter rings out across the river,
Drowning out the noise of traffic and planes,
Competing with the Angels, she is still around,
The delight which is my daughter.

Gifts of two more granddaughters arrived, one soon after Mary's death and the other five years later. Well blessed. Seven grandchildren to enjoy.

Chapter 21: Lords and Ladies

Susan Kramer was a splendid candidate in Richmond, and the Liberal Democrats were still popular nationally, the legacy of Paddy Ashdown's leadership and the deft management of the campaign – and Charles Kennedy – by the national campaign chair, Tim Razzall, a colleague from Richmond Council days who had been 'elevated' to the Lords a few years previously. Susan Kramer held my seat of Richmond Park. The LibDems gained eleven more seats with no losses. The Labour Party lost seats but retained power. The legacy of supporting the Iraq war was beginning to bite!

I retired from the House of Commons and pondered on what I would do when not helping to look after Mary's children. Too old to return to the NHS, although there were still possibilities that I could do some work in sexual and reproductive health. I did not have to ponder for long, however. One morning I received a phone call from the late Anna Werrin, Charles Kennedy's secretary of many years. She said that Charles would like me in the House of Lords! Accept a peerage? This, suggested by the man who had sacked me from the front bench for refusing to apologise to the Israel Lobby for my remarks about the Israeli government's activities in the Occupied Territories of Palestine. I expressed amazement and said I was unsure, being a firm supporter of reform of the House of Lords. Why had Charles suggested me? Anna said that I was first on his list and that his actions after my suicide bomber remarks were dictated by the party officials, not by Charles. I had always thought so. Charles was a staunch defender of human rights and international law, but I knew the restraints he was operating under, as are the leaders of all our main political groups. Subservience to the USA and its 'base' in the Middle East was paramount.

I consulted my family. Husband Keith, an NHS consultant at St Thomas' Hospital across the river, was very enthusiastic because it meant he could carry on coming across Westminster Bridge in the evenings when we were both working late and have supper together in the Terrace Café – still a favourite place for good plain food with no frills or waiters. My two sons were not keen because they thought it was going against my reforming principles, being a hypocrite in other words, and so preferred not to attend my introduction ceremony. My nephew Ted, the son of the brother who died so young, leaving me his political ambitions to fulfil, was very enthusiastic and supported me all the way. I have to admit I became enthusiastic too because it meant I could do as much or as little as I wished if the children needed me. Their other granny, Sarah Wherry, was an absolute saint for the time she gave Mary's children and the support she gave to her bereaved son, but even she needed a break each week. She is a woman in a million.

I realised that with a 'platform' in the Lords, I could go on shouting about injustice to Palestinians and the need for more emphasis on women's issues in international development. I accepted. Shirley Williams and Sally Hamwee, my old friend from Richmond Council days, were both in the Lords and agreed to introduce me in a quaint ceremony that involves wearing ermine. It was the only time I have ever worn it while taking the loyal oath in front of the whole house before processing slowly out and shaking hands with the Lord Chancellor as still was. On the way out, through a silent, packed House of Lords, a little voice was heard to shout 'Hello Nanny,' followed by muffled giggles. Mary's youngest, now three years old, disobeying orders to be quiet. It made my day.

In 2007 Gordon Brown, at last, took over from Tony Blair as Prime Minister and formed what he described as a 'government of all the talents'. Realising my left leanings and my experience in international development, I was invited, through his personal aide, Ann Keen MP, to come and talk about the possibility of joining his government and helping promote international development in the Lords as part of the Labour team there. It did not take long to decide that even though I admired Gordon Brown and his version of socialism and felt rather pleased to have been considered, I simply could not leave the Liberal Democrats after a lifetime spent in that party. I stayed on the LibDem benches until my resignation in 2016 and spent most weekends with my grandchildren and the rest of the family, trying to ensure they never felt lonely in any way.

It was good to watch Gordon Brown and Alistair Darling 'save the world' by their swift action to bail out the banks after years of loss of control of the financial sector. Sadly, it led to a huge increase in the national debt, which was used as a weapon by the Tories to attack Labour for years afterwards and led to their austerity measures. They ultimately brought divisions and unrest on the country as a whole up to and including the Brexit crisis. Strangely, the bankers in the city who had caused the crisis never suffered, and to my knowledge, never even paid more tax than the rest of us to help pay off the debt they had created.

There is much to admire in the House of Lords. Every Bill that goes through the House of Commons has a set time for scrutiny in committee. The 'guillotine' is applied, and it passes swiftly on through the remaining stages and into the House of Lords, where time is unlimited, and you begin to realise the expertise and experience in hand amongst your fellow peers. I had immediately been put on the front bench by the Leader of the LibDems in the Lords, Tom McNally, as one of two health spokespersons. The other was the hugely experienced Liz Barker. I was pleased to be doing health issues again, and I was part of our team taking the Human Embryology and Fertilisation Bill through the Lords in 2008 during that Brown 'government of all the talents'. Twice a week, we met for the committee stage of that Bill, and it was like being back at medical school in tutorials. The knowledge and expertise of Lords Darzi, Winston, Turnbull, Patel and Baroness Deech was awesome. There was great excitement during one session when a noble Lord suddenly crumpled onto the floor whilst speaking. I rushed over to him, the house was cleared, and while we waited for an ambulance Lord Darzi, the great innovative surgeon did CPR and commanded me to stay at the head end to keep our patient's airway clear. After a few minutes, our patient rose from the dead and regained consciousness. I have never forgotten the sheer delight on Ara Darzi's face when he realised his CPR was successful. He looked like a small boy, having just scrumped an apple. The peer in question was whisked away by ambulance and still attends the house most days.

It is not just scientists and lawyers who are there in abundance, but retired doctors, teachers, social workers, campaigners, architects, businessmen and women in abundance. It is those people who ultimately improve legislation – if the government approves. Any amendments passed in the Lords have to go back to the Commons, and they are often defeated there. The Commons is the elected Chamber and is the ultimate decision-maker, or rather the government whips are. This is not a justification for the unelected chamber, but a plea for more real expertise and experience before Bills are created and forced through parliament because of some manifesto commitment.

A better solution would be to replace the Lords with a 'House of Committees' where all legislation would be examined by experts co-opted for each particular Bill, before the Bill went to the Commons, during the passage of the Bill, and for a year afterwards, to see if the Bill had been as intended or needed swift revision. It would be more efficient, and certainly more economical, than having over eight hundred peers in the present House of Lords, many simply there to swell the government's chance of getting legislation through or the opposition's chance of defeating the government. The games we play. It would cease to be a luncheon and dinner venue for business peers – 'the best club in England' - as it was described by a neighbour of mine when I was sent there or 'elevated' in parliamentary terms. It has a religious note, as do the Lords Spiritual – Bishops to you and me – who are there because of history and the Anglican Church being the established church in England. Everything is because of history in our Parliament. The reason for most things is because it has always been done in that way or called a certain thing. Black Rod, for instance, is the chief executive of the House of Lords but is never referred to like that: he/she is always 'Black Rod'. But then, if we abolished or changed the House of Lords, the government of the day would lose some of its influence to garner support for its programme. Nevertheless, it must be changed eventually.

The Lords was shaken out of its complacency one afternoon in March 2017. After several terrorist attacks over the years following the invasion of Iraq, The Lord Speaker suddenly called order and stood up to announce that the chamber was being locked and we must stay on the benches until further notice. We were unable to access bags and briefcases, traditionally left on a table outside the chamber as you go in. No further information was given, and mobile phones were deployed to give us the information that there was a terrorist attack on Parliament. We knew nothing more. We stayed obediently in our places until an hour later, the doors were flung open, and four creatures resembling Star Wars characters ordered us to follow them to the Terrace Café, where we were again locked in. To our great delight, there was plenty of food and drink there. There were no staff to serve us, so with great public spirit, two Tory Baronesses leapt into action and organized a 'slate' where we could record what we were consuming to pay the next day. One of them stood guard to see fair play. After another hour or two, we were marched into the courtyard of Speaker's House, where we waited again without coats or bags until we were finally allowed to collect them. It was fairly late in the evening when we were freed by the guards who had been systematically clearing one area before moving us into it. They had checked the whole building by mid-evening and established that the terrorist was a loner. Khalid Masood had killed four people on Westminster Bridge by ramming them with his car and then had driven into the gates of the Commons Yard where he stabbed to death PC Keith Palmer before being shot dead himself.

We all trudged up to St James' Park together to get the underground home. Westminster Station was closed for the rest of that evening. A chastening experience, which will not be forgotten by MPs or Peers for a long time.

Chapter 22: Coalition Blues

Sadly, in the 2010 General Election, Gordon Brown and the Labour Party lost, but the Tories did not have an overall majority. This spelt the beginning of the end of party politics for me. After considering both options to support one or other of the main parties in coalition, the Liberal Democrats held a meeting of all peers and MPs where it was decided that we would form a coalition with the Conservatives. Nick Clegg and other senior members of our party seemed unhealthily keen to do so. Good experience and kudos for the LibDems were cited as reasons. No doubt it would be, and we were assured that a coalition agreement would be drawn up for the next five years: the fixed-term government was one of the things decided upon, as was Nick Clegg's determination to bring in Proportional Representation, which failed dismally.

We were required to betray the electorate on student tuition fees, no rise in fees having been promised during the election campaign. Students have never forgiven us for that. It was the first of many measures in that coalition government in which I voted against my party whip and did so over and over again, so disgusted was I at the agreement. No Liberal Democrat peers joined me, so trained were they even in the Lords, to obey party discipline. I argued that it would be good for the LibDem peers to vote against some of the measures agreed by the coalition and thus show the country that there were *some* good LibDems still left in the government. We could not affect the ultimate outcome, after all. I had no success. Nick Clegg led us into a very foolhardy coalition, not just because it was with the Tories – we should work with other parties – but because he gave way on so many issues dear to us, like tuition fees, in the famous 'agreement'. Worse still, he agreed to the Health and Social Care Act, which was not in the agreement nor in either party's manifesto. In fact, both parties had specifically stated that they would not do any more reorganisation of the NHS.

At the party conference that year, there was a rearguard action by the membership to try to get the leaders to change their mind about the Bill. It was felt to be such a waste of time and money and a total betrayal of the best of our public services. Astonishingly, Shirley Williams, my own and the party's 'saint', was persuaded to speak in the ensuing debate and support the coalition and the Bill. Such a sad thing to have persuaded her to do, but Shirley being Shirley, her speech swung conference and approval was given, amidst much gnashing of teeth amongst the opponents of the Bill. It is now becoming obvious that it was intended to carve up the service into nice packages to tempt the private sector to buy. As that appalling measure went through the Lords, I voted again and again against it, much to the annoyance of the Whips. Sexual and reproductive health services and family planning have gone into steep decline since they were taken over by local authorities who, cash-strapped as they are, could not see these services as a greater priority than elderly care, for example, which is one of our biggest challenges. The All-Party Group on Sexual and Reproductive Health (UK) has just produced a very worrying report on the demise of the services everyone had worked so hard to build up.

The Cameron-Clegg coalition years saw the government's wish in 2013 to support America and join the military action on Syria, which was under attack from ISIS. A brutal civil war had been started in Syria by people wanting a better life, drifting into the cities from country areas suffering drought and crop failure. A consequence of global warming, no doubt, and we are fanning the flames by our over-consumption. These people had large families to feed because there was little promotion of reproductive health and family planning outside the cities. President Assad had reacted quickly and brutally to quell the rioting and mounting unrest. Other countries became involved, led by the USA, who are always led by the Israeli government in matters concerning the Middle East, as we had already seen with the totally fabricated need to destroy Iraq years before. ISIS quickly saw an opportunity to gain territory in the ensuing chaos. To me, the Syrian civil war has always been a good example of what happens when over-consumption in the west leads to global warming, and we fail to address women's needs to reduce their family size in countries suffering drought and food shortages. It is now accepted that these factors brought together can cause massive upheavals and war. This whole subject we addressed in the paper produced by my All-Party Group entitled Population Dynamics and the Sustainable Development Goals.

The only bright light in this tragic story of the destruction of beautiful Syria, and the deaths of hundreds of thousands of its people, was the decision in the Commons for the UK *not* to support military action by the USA. The news was brought to us in the Lords by a couple of breathless MPs whilst we were debating the issue, and the nearest thing to a cheer rippled around the House of Lords. Peers do not cheer! Nevertheless, the war in Syria grinds on to a standstill, with hundreds of thousands fleeing to safety as refugees, destabilising European countries. Do the USA and its chums ever think through the consequences of their wars, apart from huge profits for the arms industries?

At the next election, the LibDems were reduced to ten seats, and Nick Clegg resigned. The price to pay for a coalition with the Tories. I was disappointed in the resignation of Nick Clegg. He had been shooed into a seat made safe by Richard Allan in Sheffield Hallam. He had not had to campaign and fight for years before becoming an MP like the rest of us. A more courageous man would have earned respect by staying on and rebuilding the party he had helped destroy. It was not to be, and the tiny rump of LibDem MPs had to start the climb all over again. They were not even the 'third' party any more. That position was held by the Scottish National Party, which had won 56 of the 59 Scottish parliamentary seats and brought some very active and interesting people into parliament. Scottish women seem to me to be much more forthright about women's issues and do not take any nonsense from the men. Particularly interesting were Philippa Whitford, a breast surgeon, who was still going out to Gaza at that time to perform life-saving surgery on the women there, and Tommy Sheppard, an ardent campaigner for the Palestinian cause. A very young woman, Mhairi Black, only twenty years old when she was elected, soon made her mark in the House of Commons with some very fiery speeches. Such a change from the pompous utterances we endured from many of the men, especially some Tories who always seem to think they have a God-given right to rule. Is it their education or what? Pomposity perfected from a very young age.

I became increasingly angry and disillusioned with my party, which I had joined formally as a fresher student in 1959, following in my father's footsteps. I took the opportunity to resign from the Liberal Democrats when they failed to give me any support on yet another Palestinian issue. My old party was no more. I was an 'Unaffiliated Peer', in the official language, confined to the misty lands of the backbenches. I quickly absorbed my new position and carried on driving the Israel Lobby mad from my new platform without having to worry about disapproval from the party managers.

Chapter 23: Chair of Pop and Sex

Without party duties, I had been able to concentrate on women's reproductive health and rights, particularly in developing countries, continuing the work I had done in the UK before I went into parliament. I remained an officer of the All-Party Parliamentary Group for Population, Development and Reproductive Health, fondly named the 'APPG for Pop and Sex' by my predecessor Christine McCafferty, Labour MP for Calder Valley. She was a hard act to follow when, in 2010, I was elected Chair of the group.

The main NGOs in this field, the United Nations Fund for Population Activities (widely known as UNFPA), the International Planned Parenthood Federation (IPPF) and Marie Stopes International (MSI), have supported this group for twenty years and provided funding for an advisor and a researcher, who have responsibility for the day to day running of the group. Our present advisor, Mette Kjaerby, is a graduate in international development. She has been in post for over ten years and, as a trained midwife with huge experience in developing countries like the Congo, is a great asset. She also possesses phenomenal energy, which puts most people to shame. The group is one of the oldest, if not the oldest, of all-party groups in parliament and has a good membership of MPs and peers from all parties and none. Our aim is to introduce as many MPs as possible to the problems faced by women in developing countries; we do this by meetings and talks and an annual study tour to show them the work being done for women's reproductive health. They come to meetings and receive briefings and suggestions for Parliamentary Questions and debates on the subject in both the Commons and the Lords. They are taken on study tours which are organised in-country by the European Forum for Population and Development and Reproductive Health and UNFPA, MSI or IPPF, who in turn are funded by philanthropists and not the taxpayer, so charges of 'another jolly' for MPs funded by the taxpayers does not apply.

It is worth repeating my mantra on women's reproductive health, which is that we are always being talked to about the 'empowerment of women', to which my response is that women cannot be empowered until they have power and control over their own bodies, and that means providing family planning services to women all over the world. Without the ability to control the number of children they have, women go on producing babies until they die. I saw this played out in abundance, even in this country, in my thirty-odd years in the NHS, where fortunately maternal deaths are not common. In developing countries, maternal death is common. The latest figure for Sierra Leone, for example, is 1,360 maternal deaths per 100,000 women. Compare that with Finland, the best country in the world in which to give birth, with a rate of 3 per 100,000 women. The UK has 9 per 100,000 women, and because of the lack of healthcare in the USA, maternal mortality is a staggering 21.6 deaths per 100,000. 'God Bless America' indeed.

The provision of family planning is such a simple and cheap intervention, and the World Economic Forum has shown that it not only benefits the women themselves, but the smaller families they have means that children get a better education and become more productive members of their society. Provision of family planning, the forum says, is the cheapest intervention we can make, which will ultimately improve the economy of a country. All of these facts have been illustrated by the late Professor Hans Rosling with his wonderful bubblegrams, which we enjoyed at conferences year after year. Despite great progress in recent years, there are still 220 million women who would use family planning if only they had access to it.

In the coalition years, the Secretary of State for International Development was Andrew Mitchell, and we secured a meeting with him early on. Andrew was always regarded as a very right-wing character and very quirky, but he had persuaded Tory MPs that international development was important, not just for the country concerned but to ensure that their increasing prosperity would benefit us too in trade agreements and fewer people to feed in crisis times. A very Tory view but effective, and it has the same outcome as the Mother Teresa approach, to help poor people in developing countries because it is the right thing to do. Both attitudes are right. Andrew was a wonderful character who greeted us at the door of his office in his socks and led us to a table where he continued to eat his sandwich lunch as we talked.

A vice-chairman of our group for some years had been Richard Ottaway, who I had fought and defeated in my council by-election in Kew many years before he became an MP. Richard was a close friend of Andrew Mitchell and a fanatic about reproductive health and family planning. They influenced each other. Andrew Mitchell was followed by the equally enthusiastic Justine Greening. This was good news all around and meant that Tory governments stuck to the aims of our group through thick and thin, despite attempts to raid the budgets during pressure from the right-wing. The situation as I write, however, is looking more ominous as the Brexit saga threatens to crash us out of the EU, led by characters like Boris Johnson and Nigel Farage and his followers, neither of whom are remotely interested in international development unless we can do trade deals with a country. Aid for trade is what it was called in the Thatcher years. The Conservatives even adopted, after pressure from Labour and LibDems, to make a firm commitment to the internationally agreed 0.7 per cent of GDP to be spent on International Development. A huge triumph for the opposition, led on this issue by the LibDems.

My speciality in women's reproductive health and family planning, much-derided when I was a doctor in the NHS, had become mainstream and a most important intervention for a developing country. Two major activities of the group, and for me in particular, are leading study tours on reproductive health to interesting countries and attending the many international conferences for parliamentarians and NGOs, often in distant and exotic places. The list is endless, and I would like to say I have truly 'visited' these cities, but conferences rarely give you the opportunity to see much. Hotels are much the same the world over, and I can never remember where we stayed. Nevertheless, for the record, I have been to and spoken at conferences in Bangkok, Kampala, Washington, New York, Ottawa, Vancouver, Paris, Kuala Lumpur, Addis Ababa. Abidjan, Stockholm, Berlin, Vienna, Athens, Bali, Copenhagen, Istanbul – and London, but I am a Londoner. Yes, I have mental pictures of these places and snatched visits after the end of the conference each day to recommended 'must visit' sights. One day maybe I can go back at leisure under my own steam and get to know them all.

I did manage to visit Vancouver with Keith years ago, and we took the 'Rocky Mountaineer' train through the mountains to Calgary, seeing a real bear on the way amongst other sights. We were extending a trip to the lakes region north of Toronto to attend a reunion of our medical year from UCH. I always have my doubts about these lavish and very expensive conferences which are held in all branches of political life. I often asked myself if the millions spent on four days in far-flung places all over the world would not be better spent on services, but then it was always argued that by going to these places, we could encourage parliamentarians from developing countries who were struggling to get women's reproductive rights in the agenda. I think, to some extent, that is true. From my perspective, if I manage to inspire a parliamentarian from a developing country to make family planning a top priority, the meeting will have been worth it. Taking Bangladesh as a good example, it is worth noting the progress that country has made since the Select Committee visited in 1999 and saw the progress of a drive on family planning. I convinced myself finally of the value of conferences when sitting alone one evening after a meal in a beach restaurant in Bali, watching the sun go down behind the volcanic mountain range across the bay. It was idyllic and so, so beautiful. I am being ironic, of course! The Gates Foundation is to be thanked for these conferences, amongst other international philanthropists – Melinda Gates is a frequent attendee.

Study tours are a different matter and pretty exhausting on the whole, along the same lines as I described earlier in detail with the Select Committee trips. Economy Class and reasonable hotels and early morning starts to visit far-flung clinics to see the progress, or not, being made by a particular country. The person who does all the logistics and sends briefings to the group members is our advisor, Mette Kjaerby. Countries visited include Malawi, Nepal, Sri Lanka, Sierra Leone and Ethiopia, with Bangladesh our most recent visit. Bangladesh is held up as a great example of family planning success for reasons I have mentioned, and we wanted to show parliamentarians how it was done. All of the study tours are funded by the European Parliamentary Forum, headed by Neil Datta, a man of many countries and none, who now lives and works in Brussels. He speaks numerous languages as he forces the subject of women's sexual and reproductive rights onto the agenda of many countries. I was President of the Forum for three years and consequently was expected to make presentations of the work of our group and 'stirring' speeches to parliamentarians from all over the world who had governments that did not want to invest in women.

One of my favourite themes to illustrate how investing in family planning ultimately improves a country's economy was to appeal to the delegates to tackle their finance ministers first – not the health ministers. Point to the wallet in his jacket and ask whether he wanted to be more affluent, and then repeat the message. Investing in family planning means smaller families, which means a better-educated workforce and prosperity for all, including the minister. It always went down well with delegates from developing countries, but when I was asked by the Guardian newspaper to talk to an invited audience about the subject not long ago, that approach was greeted with horror. How could I possibly appeal to men for women's reproductive rights? It has nothing to do with them, they argued, and I was not popular. The trouble is that after many years I have learnt that politics is 'the art of the possible', and sometimes different routes have to be taken to achieve our ends. The people from NGOs working in developing countries understood the argument, but not our idealistic feminists in the West.

A much-remembered trip was when I was invited to talk to

members of a similar group to ours in the Australian parliament in Canberra. I decided, as this was three weeks before a conference I had to attend in Bali, that I would take a holiday and do a little self-funded, lone exploration of Australia on my way back to Bali. The meeting was disrupted by it being the first Prime Minister's Questions session of the new parliament, and Malcolm Turnbull was the new Prime Minister. I was led to the front row of the visitors' gallery and even welcomed courteously by the Speaker of the Parliament. I watched whilst Turnbull comprehensively demolished Bill Shorten, the Labor leader, who had decided to attack Turnbull because the new Prime Minister and his wife were wealthy lawyers. Malcolm Turnbull was convincingly honest and asked what was wrong with getting rich by honest hard work with all taxes paid? It was a masterclass in Prime Minister's answers, but, like all Australian Prime Ministers, he did not last long, and now Australia is in the grips of the right-wing, which seems to be sweeping the world.

I visited friends in Sydney, Adelaide and Perth on that trip, and a visit to a project for Aboriginal women up in Alice Springs was also interesting but depressing. They seemed so far away from our culture. At Uluru (Ayers Rock), I learned some of the legends of the indigenous people and wondered how on earth they could be truly integrated. It is not just language and development. Theirs is a different mindset altogether from ours. Nevertheless, we must try. As with the Kalahari Bushmen and the First People of North America, it seemed almost too late to try to integrate them. What damage have we wrought in this world of ours in the name of progress? On the other hand, at the Alice Springs original Telegraph Station, I learned the truly awe-inspiring story of how pioneers, helped by camels, managed to put a telephone line across Australia from Darwin to Adelaide in the 19th century. There is a small museum at that Telegraph Station, recording how Aboriginal children were taken away from their parents and 'placed' with white Australian families for education and to be 'civilised'. They were mostly treated as slaves. All progress? Recently with catastrophic fires raging in New South Wales and Victoria, Australians have looked again at the skilled land management of the Aboriginals, which the colonists so disregarded. They had a lot of experience and skill to offer, which was swept aside in the rush to acquire land for the great British Empire.

I then had an extra week in Perth caught by the volcano clouds of dust emanating from the Bali volcano, which caused our conference there to be postponed until the following January. No aeroplanes could fly, and my energy-saving scheme to help the planet was wrecked. The best-laid plans …….

Chapter 24: The Great Abortion Debate

A major problem for all of us working in women's reproductive health is the attitude to abortion of the Catholic Church and at the other end of the Christian spectrum, the Evangelicals, especially in America, which is the biggest aid donor in the world. Those Evangelical Christians in the United States of America are totally against abortion at any stage and, because presidents of that country depend on their support financially, and in voter turnout, American aid policy under George W. Bush and now Donald Trump has been against abortion. Any aid programme that may include advice about, or the provision of, safe abortion is shunned. That effectively means all aid from the USA for women's reproductive health is stopped. Bush introduced what was referred to as the 'Gag' Rule, which forbade any development funds to go to NGOs which provided abortion. This was a very serious move, and it stopped many programmes in their tracks because abortion, or even abortion counselling, was bound to be included at some stage in the provision of healthcare for women. Somehow progress was still made during those years with other countries stepping up their provision of aid and with the intervention of some individual donors. The situation was eased somewhat in the Obama years, although not encouraged, such is the electoral consequence of offending the evangelical movement. When Donald Trump came into power in America, the situation worsened to the extent that even NGOs who may have contact with other NGOs, who may only advise on abortion, were banned from receiving US aid. The situation is being likened to *The Handmaid's Tale* by Margaret Atwood, which was made into a popular and very frightening TV drama. The US administration, apparently, likes women's bodies to be controlled by men. The choice was gone, and the consequence for women in developing countries was more deaths from unsafe, botched abortions and more unwanted children. Once more, the international community is having to scrape around to try to make up the deficit in funding for women's reproductive health.

For women within the USA, however, where they had fought for and got abortion rights, it means that there are regular attacks, legal and otherwise, on the abortion laws. Various anti-abortion laws have been in force in each state since at least 1900. The US Supreme Court decriminalised abortion nationwide in 1973, in a case described as 'Roe v. Wade'. Abortion was already legal in several states, but the decision imposed a uniform framework for federal legislation on the subject. This ruling is so precious to American women and needs to be defended. Defend it they do, against constant picketing of clinics where abortion may be part of the services provided and attacks on doctors who do the operation. One doctor was shot dead outside his clinic.

Whatever one's personal attitude to abortion may be, and many books have been written on the subject, I firmly contend that it is a woman's right to choose what she does with her own body. Only she can judge her personal and family circumstances. Religion should not come into it. If others think abortion is a sin, then it is for a woman to decide whether she 'sins' or not. As a medic who knows how many fertilised eggs never actually attach to the lining of the uterus and so are wasted naturally, I cannot see the religious arguments either. I remember a bishop speaking in the House of Lords on one occasion and relating how Victorian clerics agonised about this and thought abortion was a sin once the soul had entered the foetus. The problem then is when does this occur? They determined at one stage that it was 12 weeks for the male foetus and 16 weeks for the female foetus, to which a feminist wag responded, 'Ah yes, when God made man, She was only testing.' The other argument that irritates, and indeed amuses, is when some opponent of abortion asked how I would have felt if I had been aborted and not allowed to live, which is the most ridiculous comment of all. If I did not exist, how on earth would I be able to comment on my non-existence? What is their problem?

When I was a junior hospital doctor, before the Abortion Act of

1967 so brilliantly piloted through parliament by David Steel, I saw women who had been to illegal abortionists or tried to do it themselves: the suffering was intense, physically and emotionally. In developing countries, unsafe abortion is the major cause of maternal death. Desperate women adopt desperate measures like coat-hangers, soapy douches, syringes – anything that might dislodge the unwanted pregnancy – and all methods risk sepsis, chronic illness, or death. It is not widely known that abortion rates are roughly the same in countries where it is legally available and countries where it is banned – roughly 34 abortions per 1000 women of childbearing age – but, in those countries where abortion is banned, 68,000 women die every year from unsafe abortion, so desperate is their situation when they discover they are pregnant.

Another aspect of this harrowing subject is the battle that wages over abortion after rape in conflict situations. You would think that this would be a 'given' and that it would be available, but there are long battles about the subject, and the US administration will not even allow that. In international law, however, it is part of a woman's reproductive right to have an abortion after rape in conflict, but American NGOs and their partners are forbidden to perform them. It is hard to imagine the suffering and anguish of a woman in a war zone who has been repeatedly raped, sometimes in front of her children, and brutally, not just simple sexual intercourse, having then to endure a pregnancy. Fortunately, in some areas of conflict, especially where our own and European NGOs operate, this service is available, but it is all very much under wraps, for the women's sake as much as the NGOs. Talking to women in refugee camps fleeing war, the overwhelming impression I get is their shame at such a thing happening to them and fear, in many cases, that their husbands will turn them out of the family home if they ever return and the husbands find out. It is still so common for women to be blamed for rape, even if it was gang rape by soldiers at gunpoint. Such is the position of women in some places in the twenty-first century.

Abortion law varies all over the world. In Canada, for example, they have one of the most liberal abortion laws in the world, it being legal at all stages of pregnancy to be dealt with as a medical matter between doctor and patient. Of course, in some parts of Canada, access is difficult because of distances, but nevertheless, that country stands as a shining example to the rest of the world. On the other hand, the law in El Salvador is so strict that there are currently women in prison who have had miscarriages naturally and have been accused by someone or other that they have procured an abortion.

As I have mentioned before, Bangladesh stands out as a country, not only because it has been promoting family planning ever since the time, in the seventies, when Sheik Rahman, the present Prime Minister's father, was in power. He was assassinated and is now regarded as a national hero. Bangladesh has officially 'compromised' and allowed 'menstrual regulation' for decades, even though 'abortion' is illegal in that country. It is worth remembering that menstrual regulation is how they describe abortion up to nine weeks, medically or surgically.

Most countries come somewhere in between these two extremes. The UK should be updating its own Abortion Act. It is currently allowed up to 24 weeks if the mental or physical health of the mother would be affected if she continues with the pregnancy. There is no limit on abortion for a severely handicapped foetus or if the mother's life is at risk. It is sad that two doctors' signatures are required before an abortion can occur, which in the present state of the NHS can cause a delay. Without fulfilling these conditions, abortion is still a criminal act under the Offences Against the Person Act of 1861. This all needs updating, and efforts are made from time to time to do this. I tabled a Private Member's Bill to make two doctors' signatures unnecessary, but the government did not 'find time' for it. Neither did the government find time for a Private Member's Bill to exclude the severe handicap of a foetus from the reasons for an abortion, on the grounds that it was discriminatory to handicapped people and foetuses. Currently, efforts are being made to decriminalise abortion and make it part of health care, which is how it is handled in Canada. This would seem the best solution but, with all the changes in government recently, will it find a slot somewhere? There would then remain the thorny problem of doctors who conscientiously object to abortion on religious grounds, for which I have no patience. There are countless specialities one can choose from as a junior doctor, and there is no need to go for a speciality where you would not take part in an essential part of women's healthcare.

There has been one success recently in Northern Ireland. MPs in the women's health group tabled an amendment to the Northern Ireland (Executive Formation) Bill. The government in Northern Ireland had been suspended for two years with no resolution in sight. The amendment was to decriminalise abortion and allow same-sex marriage, both measures fiercely resisted by the DUP, the politicians who at that time had the majority in Northern Ireland. In the Republic of Ireland, after a referendum massively in favour of decriminalising abortion, the law was changed. The women of Northern Ireland deserve the same treatment. There are even women there who are awaiting prosecution for obtaining abortion pills on the internet for very early medical abortion. The House of Lords sat until after midnight to ensure this Bill would become law, against fierce opposition from what I can only call some very bigoted people who want to impose their religious beliefs on others. They failed, and the law came into force this October 2019. The amendment to the Northern Ireland (Executive Formation) Act delivers long-awaited abortion law reform, including decriminalisation. This will stop women from being prosecuted for accessing abortion and introduce a suspension for current cases.

My long-term dream for women, who for their own reasons cannot or do not want to be pregnant, and cannot face the physical and social changes an unwanted pregnancy imposes, is for the medical abortion pill, which can be taken safely up to 12 weeks, to become legally available at pharmacies, and the whole ritual of seeing doctors and getting permission becomes a thing of the past, much as the 'morning-after pill' has become. I understand it happens in Pakistan, albeit under the radar at present. I predict that abortion will take the form of a 'late period pill' in much the same way as the morning-after pill is now accepted. I want my granddaughters to be free to do what they want with their own bodies. That is empowerment!

Chapter 25: FGM and Other Abuses

When I was practising in Southall in the1980s, I had a lovely Somali patient. She was a student in London and had come to ask for a smear test and advice on contraception. That is how she introduced herself, and I duly went through the options with her. She was insistent on me doing a vaginal examination, which I did not normally do unless the patient requested it. She was very insistent, and when I looked at her, I genuinely did not know what I was looking at. She told me that she had been 'cut' as a small child and wanted to know whether anyone could help her. That was my first experience of a patient who had had the cruel practice of Female Genital Mutilation – FGM – performed on her as a small child, without anaesthetic or any sterile equipment. She had had her clitoris and inner labia removed and the whole vulva stitched up to leave one small hole for both urine and menstruation to pass through. That university student opened up a huge area of women's health care that was not known to many of us. It presented problems for this girl who genuinely wanted to be made 'normal' again, but it also opened up huge problems for obstetric departments when more Somali women escaping the war were treated in our hospitals. Apparently, if the 'hole' is too small for sexual intercourse on the wedding night, the husband cuts it open to allow penetration. That hole, once healed, is not big enough for the baby's head at delivery, so more surgery is needed, and then even more intervention afterwards, as some women demanded to be sewn up again so their husbands would not complain.

When I got into parliament, this had become quite a topic, as more and more refugees came to us from Somalia. As early as 1983, the practice had been made illegal in the UK, but the group thought that an in-depth investigation should be undertaken and more powerful legislation introduced to stop girls from being taken abroad for the procedure. Ruth Rendell, in the House of Lords, famous as a crime writer, was a tireless campaigner to end the practice. Ann Clwyd introduced a Bill in the Commons, which I sponsored. It is now well recognised, and teachers, doctors, nurses and social workers are all trained to spot any signs that a girl may be going 'abroad' in the school holidays. Staff at the airports have also been alerted to look out for likely cases.

A few years ago, a colleague and I, on a flight out to a conference in Addis Ababa at the beginning of the school summer holidays, thought it strange that there seemed to be very few men on the flight, mainly women and girls. The flight to Addis connected with a flight to Mogadishu in Somalia. When we were able, we reported this to the Home Office, which now has a special unit dealing with the subject. No prosecutions ensued on that occasion, however, but how could we be sure that none of those girls had had FGM whilst abroad? It is so difficult because the girls themselves will not testify against their mothers and grandmothers, who have made them believe it was for their own 'good'. Fortunately, it is now not necessary to have the child's evidence. If FGM has been inflicted on a child, then the adult responsible for the child must be prosecuted.

Despite all the efforts of campaigners and professionals and the changes made to educate everyone in touch with women and girls, we are very slow to make progress in the form of prosecutions. LibDem MP Lynne Featherstone, as International Development Minister, did sterling work on this during the coalition government. Eventually, only education and assimilation with other cultures will stop this horrible practice, which not only causes ill health and sometimes death, but when the full procedure is done, it denies the girl any sexual pleasure all her life. Most authorities on the subject say this is why it was done in the ancient past so that women would not enjoy sex and so stay faithful to their man. The men wanted girls to have FGM so that they could be sure of complete control over their women. It is not a religious practice and not linked to any particular culture or religion, but it prevails in many African countries as far apart as Somalia and Sierra Leone and also parts of the Middle East. Egypt, strangely, despite having a law against it, has a high incidence of FGM.

I have wondered for a long time whether it was always done so that men could have 'control' of their women. Or could it have been a health measure, as is always claimed of male circumcision? I am shouted down by the campaigners. Will we ever know the origins of FGM? It is still practised and, certainly in modern times, has a mission to control women and make them more 'desirable' to men. It is abhorrent, and so is male circumcision, in my opinion, unless there are real medical indications. That does not make me popular with some religious groups. There are so many different groups now campaigning on different aspects of FGM, some even in this country, promoting it as a traditional practice that is 'harmless' and hating the government here for intervening in their lives. To venture into this argument needs lots of courage and a very resilient personality. Supporters of the practice, and there are plenty, argue that it is a cultural tradition and that we have no business interfering with such matters. But ducking stools and the burning of witches were once cultural traditions in this country that thankfully are no longer practised. Once again, it is my experience with actual patients and the consequences of the practice which drives me on.

All over the world, where the APPG has gone on study tours, we have seen the horrors of child marriage, defined internationally in the 'Rights of the Child' as marriage before the age of 18. We decided in 2012 to do an investigation into the subject, with hearings taken from experts and victims, followed by a report. There has been much concern in this country over girls, mainly from the Indian subcontinent, being sent home to be married, and we heard evidence of such cases from the women themselves. It is important to distinguish between child marriage and forced marriage. Child marriage is almost always forced marriage, but forced marriage is not always child marriage, so it is important to tread carefully. It is also important to distinguish between forced marriage and 'arranged' marriages, many of which are just helpful parents introducing their children to suitable boys or girls until something clicks and they agree. Many such marriages are very happy – or as happy as most. Jasvinder Sanghera was a victim herself, being forced by her parents to be married to a person she would only meet on her wedding day. She refused and escaped from the family, only to have been ostracised by them ever since. Her sister's story is even more harrowing and ended in her suicide. Jasvinder did, however, found a thriving organisation called 'Karma Nirvana', which helps many children being coerced into marriage. Her book *Shame* and subsequent writings are well worth reading. She is now a CBE, rewarding her efforts for victims, but the battle continues.

During the group's investigation, we heard of many such stories here in the UK and abroad. The one I remember most vividly was a case in Afghanistan where a twelve-year-old girl was forced to marry a man in his sixties. On her wedding night, he was so brutal that she died of a severe haemorrhage the following morning. Her wedding day picture adorns the cover of 'A Childhood Lost', our group's paper on the subject. All over the world, despite national laws to stop the practice, girls are being married too early, often for a good dowry, or because their parents fear they will be raped if they are not 'safe' with a husband.

Quite recently, I took a break in Jordan with a good friend Salwar Amor who worked helping to make documentaries for Channel Four, most recently in Syria. During a great week, including a long day driving to see Petra, we spent time with the refugees in the huge Zaatari Camp. I was told that mothers would prefer to marry their daughters to someone they knew, but, in the camp surroundings, the fear of rape was so great that girls as young as twelve were being found husbands who they had to marry. Those mothers were doing it to protect their daughters. What has the world come to? Of course, it has always been like this before mass media and the internet exposed these practices.

We had our own struggle in parliament after our report was finished because, although the internationally accepted age of marriage is 18, the UK, which gives aid to projects all over the world to prevent child marriage, still allows marriage at 16 – with parental consent. Interesting that during the debate when I introduced an amendment to another Bill to raise the age of marriage to 18, one noble Lord said it had to be 16 because if a girl got pregnant even in our society, it would be a shame on her family unless she could be married. I could hardly believe my ears in 2019. Others supported the government line that 16 should be upheld, providing the parents consented and that their consent was witnessed by someone of their religion. How naive is that? If a girl or boy is terrified of going against their parent's wishes, won't they automatically say they agree? The stupidity of governments – or is it a desire not to offend certain groups of voters?

We shall try again.

Chapter 26: Better off Dead

World authorities talk at length about the maternal mortality rate (MMR). It is coming down since we have been concentrating on reproductive health and family planning worldwide. In the early 1990s, 385,000 women died in childbirth every year, which is like two jumbo jets carrying approximately 500 passengers crashing every day of the year. That surely would create headlines? By introducing better maternal care in many countries and making access to family planning easier, this figure has reduced to 216,000. A 44 per cent decrease is worth having, and it must go on getting better.

There is a problem, however. I have long pointed out that measuring MMR is all very well, but what about the maternal morbidity rate – that is, the women who are physically and sometimes mentally damaged by childbirth because of lack of care. At first, no one was particularly interested – they will cope within the family, I was told. The truth is quite different, and I persuaded the APPG to investigate this subject because, as far as I was concerned, a woman who is badly damaged in childbirth is often rejected by her husband and family and might be better off dead. The phrase stuck and became the title of our report. 'Better off Dead' was snapped up at every conference we went to and is the only report by the group to have run out of hard copies. Forgive me for one last 'brag'. The then President of the Royal College of Obstetricians and Gynaecologists told me he took our report all over the world and often referred to it. The group was proud of that, and so was I, although I don't do 'proud' because it usually comes before a fall. Let us say I was pleased.

The most dramatic injury we saw after childbirth was the fistula, when a passageway is torn between the bladder, vagina and rectum. In Nepal, Ethiopia and Sierra Leone, which we visited, they were trying to help women suffering from fistula. We heard story after story. If labour is very long, usually because the baby is in the wrong position, women in developing countries may have to travel long distances to get help. We heard of women in labour in Nepal travelling a day or more on a donkey, led by a relative over hills and mountains to get help from a doctor. Help is invariably too late, and either mother and baby are dead on arrival, or the baby is dragged out or delivered, leaving permanent damage to the mother. In many cultures, childbirth is made much more dangerous by the practice of FGM and child marriage. Holes open up between the vagina and bladder, colon or rectum, allowing a flow of urine and faeces via the vagina to the outside. The woman has no control over it all and has no sanitary protection such as women in the west might use. She becomes smelly, and her family rejects her. Some women leave the family home completely; others we heard were confined in a shed away from the main living space, sometimes with the animals. This condition is much more likely to happen in young girls who are not physically mature enough to give birth to babies but have been victims of child marriage. We already knew that in some cultures, women were not allowed to be in the main living quarters of the family or to prepare food for them when menstruating and would be confined to sheds once a month if they were lucky enough not to be permanently pregnant! A terrible life of suffering for them.

On the brighter side, we saw two wonderful hospitals where these girls were being helped. In Ethiopia, girls and women with fistula were first recognised by Dr Catherine Hamlin and her husband Reginald, Australian gynaecologists, who resolved to set up a hospital just outside Addis Ababa where these girls and women could be treated. Catherine Hamlin went on to set up five more regional hospitals in Ethiopia to treat fistula. Her hospital outside Addis Ababa is a wonderful place, on a hill outside the city, with clean wards and hopeful, cheerful patients who may have travelled alone for days to get there for help. After they have been treated, they are given fresh clothes and encouraged to return to their families if the family will have them.

We also heard of girls who were trained as operating theatre technicians to do the simpler operations themselves and so increase the number of patients treated. Doctors from all over the world go to Addis to see the Hamlins' work and train in their techniques. On my first visit, I was able to meet Catherine Hamlin, who was then in her eighties and still working and encouraging these girls and women to start their lives afresh. It is all financed by charitable donations, and treatment is free. Inspirational stuff for those who can access it. The hospitals aim to cure 4000 women annually, but Catherine Hamlin cited the World Health Organisation's estimate that there were 6000-7000 cases a year in Ethiopia alone. Twice nominated for the Nobel Peace Prize, she died aged 97 in 2020.

In Freetown, Sierra Leone, another centre, called the Aberdeen Women's Hospital, was set up by Ann Gloag, a founder of the transport company Stagecoach. It is supported by UNFPA and delivers 3000 babies a year, as well as repairing fistula and rehabilitating the young women. Children's services, including vaccination, are also offered. It is a very bright facility in an otherwise desperately poor Sierra Leone, one of the poorest countries in the world, and then still suffering the Ebola outbreak ten years after the war ended there. The good news is that these services are spreading worldwide, and our own Royal College of Obstetrics and Gynaecology is promoting projects in Nepal, Tanzania and Uganda.

Another condition that affects women in our societies is prolapse of the uterus and weakness of the vaginal wall after childbirth, which can cause rectal and bladder prolapse. All these conditions are treatable in the west. The difference for women in poorer countries is that there is little treatment available. They have to live with it, likewise severe anaemia due to post-partum haemorrhage, poor nutrition and high blood pressure following eclampsia in pregnancy, if they are lucky enough to survive. Terrible infections are common in developing countries after childbirth – the 'puerperal fever' which haunted mothers in the west too before antibiotics became available; because of this infection, many babies were left motherless. I could have been such a baby during the Second World War, but my mother recovered thank goodness.

Even AIDS, which despite huge efforts by the drug companies and governments worldwide to eradicate the disease, still stalks the continent of Africa and affects women more than men because our anatomy is so vulnerable. Women of indigenous people all over the world are particularly vulnerable to malnutrition and disease, as it becomes more and more impossible to live their traditional lifestyles mainly because of the march of Europeans, who have invaded their lands and used them to extract our modern western needs. We are responsible for global warming too, which is causing desertification and wars and migration of people to other lands for a better life. We have the nerve to grumble about immigrants and asylum seekers—shame on us all.

Battles there are still to be fought until women and their families all over the world have the same chances in life as we do.

Chapter 27: Epilogue

I am now approaching the end of my days and will soon be hanging up my parliamentary pass and starting to do retired things. Keith spent his working life as a neuroradiologist at St Thomas' Hospital, a far cry from his farming family roots in Dorset. He died at the age of 71, a good biblical innings by our family standards but, of course, so sad for us all. He was much loved. I moved again, to a third-floor flat overlooking Kew village through two magnificent oak trees which chart the months passing and provide endless amusement with spats going on between the indigenous English birds and those cheeky colonising parakeets trying to take their territory, a constant reminder of the Israeli settlers in the West Bank of Palestine. I can see the world come and go and contemplate the future, such as it is. My grandchildren are all doing well, and Mary's boys have done their mother proud. Keith would love to know that they are both at university and enjoying life. After such a shock in their childhood years, this grandmother did worry, but perhaps it spurred them on in the same way that young Palestinians strive to do better and better in education against all odds for when their liberation comes?

Before I do retire, however, and get too complacent, the world has been taken by storm, and normal life has ceased, for we do not know how long. Shortly after I returned from a holiday of a lifetime in New Zealand and Australia with my eldest son, returning via Beijing, and after a very jolly Christmas seeing all the family, news reports started coming through about a new type of virus inelegantly named COVID-19, which had emerged in Wuhan in China. It rapidly spread across the world, and by February of 2020, it was declared a pandemic, and a very deadly one, attacking older people and the already sick disproportionately. Consequently, 'the crumblies', as I like to call us, are locked down in our homes, lest we catch the virus and become a burden on the NHS by taking up beds needed for younger, more productive members of our society. A wise decision. Whole families were told to stay at home and only emerge for brief exercise sessions and food shopping. Shops, pubs, restaurants, and all places where people gather were closed down.

We are now eight weeks into the lockdown. Schools and universities have remained closed and teach what they can over the internet. Families make frantic plans about food and essential supplies. Unaccountably, the supermarkets first ran out of toilet rolls, leading to lots of ribaldry on social media and radio and television, and very soon after ran out of many other supplies, essential and less essential, most seriously a desperate shortage quickly became apparent of essential protective equipment needed for frontline workers fighting the pandemic. As the seriousness of our situation has sunk in, the laughing has stopped, and I have to look forward to more weeks, if not months, of isolation. I wish that I could abandon politics and my old age and go to help colleagues in the National Health Service. The NHS has been run down by ten years of Tory government and simply did not have the beds or equipment to cope at first, which, as someone who had opposed the Coalition Government's so-called reforms and angered the Liberal Democrat whips by doing so, has made me very angry. It looked at first like the service would be overwhelmed until plans were laid for new 'fever' hospitals named after one of my heroines Florence Nightingale. Essential supplies such as protective clothing and masks had to be obtained, in competition with countries all over the world needing the same things.

My world has shrunk, and I think of those early postwar years of my childhood, with food rationing and with activities limited. One of the most striking similarities is the silence of the streets, with the occasional car or bicycle passing by. The streets are so quiet that early one morning, I watched as a boy on his bicycle joyfully hurtled up the main road doing 'wheelies' all the way. The peace is disturbed from time to time by ambulances wailing as they take stricken patients to the hospital, evoking memories of air raid warning sirens, which were used by factories in the Black Country long after the war ended, marking the end of shifts for their workers.

Heathrow Airport is almost closed down, and instead of the continual roar of aeroplanes overhead, you can hear the birds singing their hearts out. I even found myself one day running to the window when I heard an aeroplane, just as we children did in the forties and fifties when they were still a rare sight. I had an even greater sense of déjà vu when a friend rang me up to say that our local shop had pasta if I could not get it anywhere else – fortunately, I prefer good old English spuds to pasta. My mother and her sisters were always tipping each other off when something became available in our local shops after the war. Instead of making children's clothes out of almost anything, women at home with sewing machines are making protective gowns for the young people on the front line. Face masks are being made too, but not nearly as sophisticated as my Mickey Mouse gas mask, which I had during the war. I was sad when it had to go back, unworn, to the War Office.

The great battle of the COVID-19 Virus is on, and the doctors, nurses and other NHS staff do not flinch. Neither do the carers, truck and van, bus and train drivers, shopkeepers, till operators, refuse collectors and masses of other people, often low paid and disregarded in our modern society, who have become our pandemic heroes. They keep society going, often risking their own lives in the process. In the First World War, our young soldiers were cannon fodder as wave after wave of them gave up their lives in the trenches. In the Second World War, young men and women were sacrificed to save our way of life. Now the young are fighting a deadly foe that threatens our livelihoods and our society. We have much to be thankful for and many people to be grateful to.

The women once again are at home. Some are working online. Many are acting as teachers for different age children and providing peace and quiet when possible for fathers also working at home. They are shopping and cooking for family and neighbours who cannot go out, and in my daughter-in-law's case studying for a higher degree at the same time as juggling everything else. Other women are struggling to cope with children in high-rise flats or temporary accommodation, some with violent partners from whom there is no escape. The women, as ever, are showing how to keep society together. I am one of the lucky ones. I only have to stay locked up.

The Prime Minister has been in intensive care with the infection. He has now recovered and has to try and convince us all that this situation will go on for a long time if we are finally to eradicate this virus from our lives. Nobody has any real idea how long it will take, and daily bulletins on new cases and deaths keep us informed of progress should there be any—a strange way to end a life.

'Will I survive longer than the virus,' is a question many elderly people are asking themselves.

When I look back to that little girl, standing in the smoke from train engines at the top of our road in the Black Country and dreaming of her future, I certainly never dreamed of all this. Throughout my time in medicine and politics, as I have already indicated, I have heard the words 'empowerment of women' bandied about by politicians, usually men. They think that by saying it and experimenting with quotas for women in politics and management, the problem will resolve itself. Many countries of the world, including my beloved Palestine, need more action from its women, bowed down by poverty and childbearing.

I became a member of parliament after twenty years of being a local activist, a councillor, a doctor and a mother of three. It took a long time and a lot of effort and support. In developing countries, women and girls are not so lucky. It is why our government and others have focused on this aspect of overseas aid in recent years and why my 'Cinderella' speciality of family planning, which I chose to pursue way back in the 1960s, is now such an important topic. It has worked to the advantage of the developed world, too, improving economies and giving us more trading partners eventually. This is the chief reason why I suspect it is espoused by my political opponents. World population growth is endangering the planet by creating too many people on too little land in poor countries and too many consumers creating global warming in the West. It is madness not to address this by being serious about climate change but also being serious about universal free family planning. Do not ever refer to birth control. That implies coercion which there should never be. Voluntary family planning is the preferred term always.

I remember the delight I felt in July 2012 walking up to the Queen Elizabeth II Conference Centre opposite Westminster Abbey and seeing a huge banner proclaiming 'FAMILY PLANNING 2020' – then eight years in the future. It was a conference called by our government and financed mainly by the Bill and Melinda Gates Foundation. My humble insistence over the years, in the Midlands and London, that family planning was as important an intervention as any other medical speciality, had won support. I wanted all those medical colleagues to see that banner and attend that conference. They who had teased the doctor who eschewed fame in the medical hierarchy to help train other doctors, yes registrars in obstetrics too, in the methods and techniques available and help build up a Faculty of Sexual and Reproductive Health.

I suppose though if I had an apotheosis – you know, when the light shines and happiness is all around, and our hero floats upwards to paradise – it was when I heard, during that working holiday in Australia, that 'I' had been made a Fellow of the Royal College of Obstetricians and Gynaecologists (Honoris Causa) for the work that had been done for women in the UK and developing countries. It was not just for me, which I made clear in my acceptance speech, but for the members of my group and our advisor, Mette Kjaerby, who had worked so hard to promote women's reproductive rights in many ways. It was a huge collective effort. The award was for the All-Party Parliamentary Group, not just me.

It would have pleased my mother even more than hearing me on 'Any Questions'.

Promoting women's reproductive health is not just good for women's empowerment, and ultimately the prosperity of their countries, but it is the right thing to do. Whatever the other arguments, women have reproductive rights. We are the producers of the next generation, and we also happen to have the same intelligence and brains as men, albeit, some would argue, in different fields. We should be allowed to have a life that is *not* just having children until we die.

My parents gave me the encouragement I needed. My teachers at school and university gave me the skills. My colleagues in the medical profession made sure I was fit and well enough to continue my work on many occasions, and my dear family and friends gave me the support and love to plough on through the difficult times. I thank them all, but I want to remind them all, constantly, that women want opportunities, not to compete with men but to work equally alongside them.

It is worth remembering Mary Wollstonecraft, an early feminist, who said,

'I do not wish women to have power over men, but over themselves.'

Indeed so.

Acknowledgements

My husband, the late Dr Keith Tonge, for his patience, forbearance and sense of humour over the years.

My parents, who gave me every opportunity in life. The headteacher of Dudley Girls' High School, the late Mary Ambrose who was a role model in how to deal with adversity.

My children and grandchildren for giving me so much love and pleasure, and for putting up with me.

Jake Wherry, my son in law, who has faced so many crises in his life but has remained steady and supportive of his boys and a staunch friend, and kept us on our toes with his band 'Herbalizer'

Caroline Blomfield, my dear friend, advisor and sometime critic and editor.

Louise Arimatsu who with David Williams and others won the Richmond Park seat for us in 1997 with their brilliant strategy and literature .

Mette Kjaerby, Advisor to my All-Party Parliamentary Group., and Myfanwy Probyn, the group's researcher, for keeping me focused on women's reproductive health and rights whatever else was being thrown at me.

Sally Fitzharris, journalist and friend who has encouraged me to write this book and helped so much with editing
.

Miranda Pinch, campaigner, filmmaker and researcher whose energy never flags.

Past Presidents of the RCOG, for the help they have given to the All Party Parliamentary Group on Population, Development and

Reproductive Health.

Richmond Park Liberal Democrats and the late David Blomfield, who with David Williams, Serge Lourie and Gareth Roberts, with their years of hard work, have retained the parliamentary seat of Richmond Park for the Liberal Democrats

My office staff in Richmond: Serena Hennessey, Nick Carthew, the late Polly Wright and Andrew Pilkington, who were always ready to do the extra hour and protected me on many occasions.

My researchers in the House of Commons, especially the inspirational Vanessa Haines and Alice Hutchinson.

The '59ers of UCL/H, my medical student friends, who have stayed together over many decades.

The medical and nursing staff in Women's Services in Ealing and especially Doreen Burchett, whose enthusiasm for women's health was an inspiration.

My colleagues and friends everywhere, without whose love and encouragement I would not be here today.

Valentina Rinaldi for the cover design which has given me such pleasure and brought back many memories.

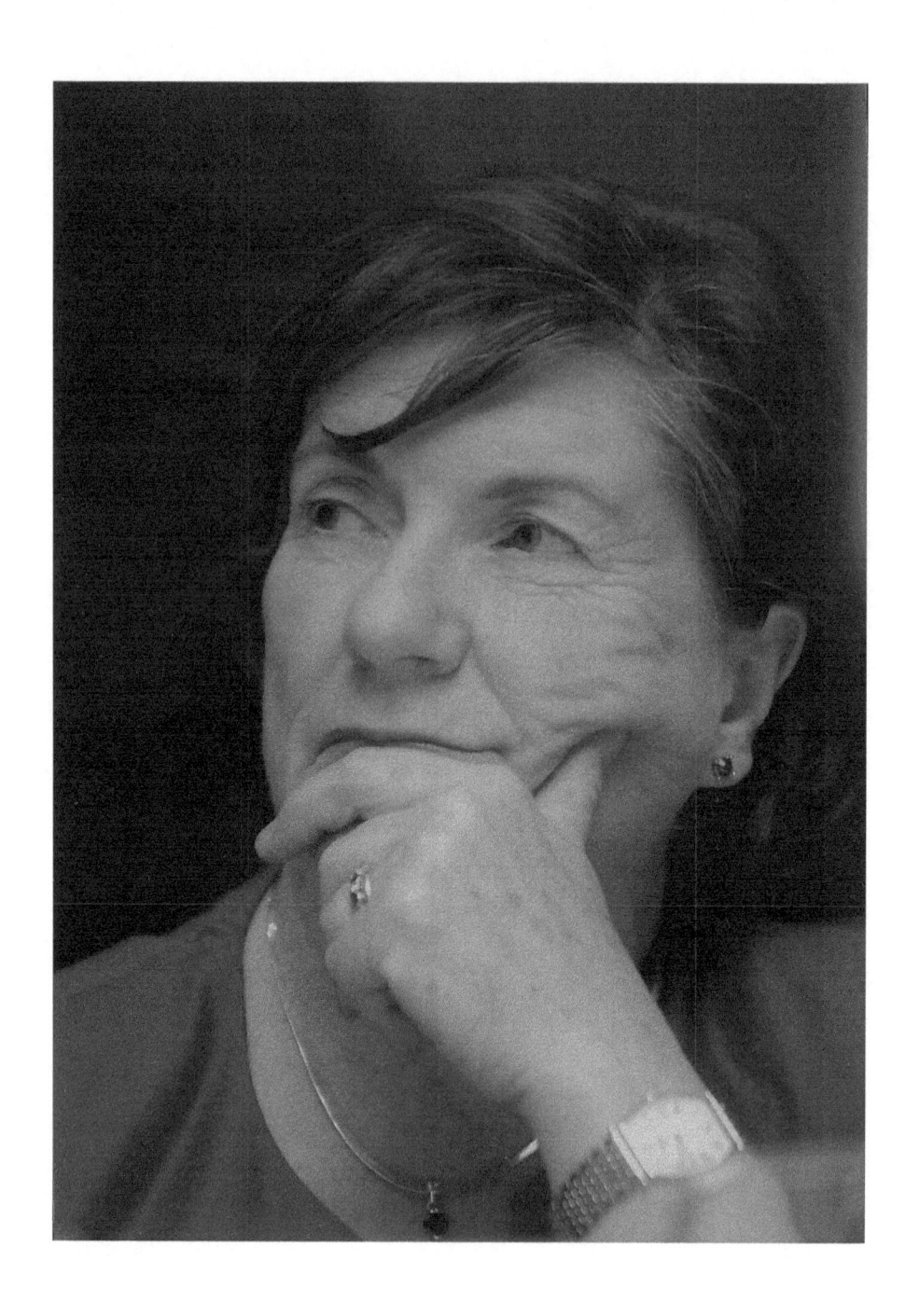

Jenny Tonge

Jenny graduated as a medical doctor from University College London in 1964. Subsequently, she worked for over 30years in the NHS, her speciality being sexual and reproductive health and women's health care.

After eight years as a local councillor in the London Borough of Richmond upon Thames, she was elected to parliament in 1997 as MP for Richmond Park.

She stood down from the House of Commons in 2004 after her daughter was killed in an electrical accident, leaving two small boys. The following year, she was offered a life peerage in recognition of her work as the Lib Dem Shadow Secretary of State for International Development and entered the House of Lords as Baroness Tonge of Kew.

She continued her interest in international development in the Lords, in parallel with women's health in developing countries.

As Chair of the all-party group for Population Development and Reproductive Health, she put pressure on the Department for International Development to make family planning a top priority, which it became.

She first became interested in the Palestine/Israel issue during a visit to Israel and the occupied territories of Palestine (including Gaza) in 2003, which she described as 'a life-changing experience'.

Since then, she has been an outspoken and controversial figure for her continuing support of the Palestinian people and her frank criticism of the Israeli government.